The Heart
Healthy Diet
for Two

1500 Days of Simple and Wholesome Dishes with a 28-Day Meal Plan for Two Hearts to Enjoy | Full Color Edition

Polly R. Pendleton

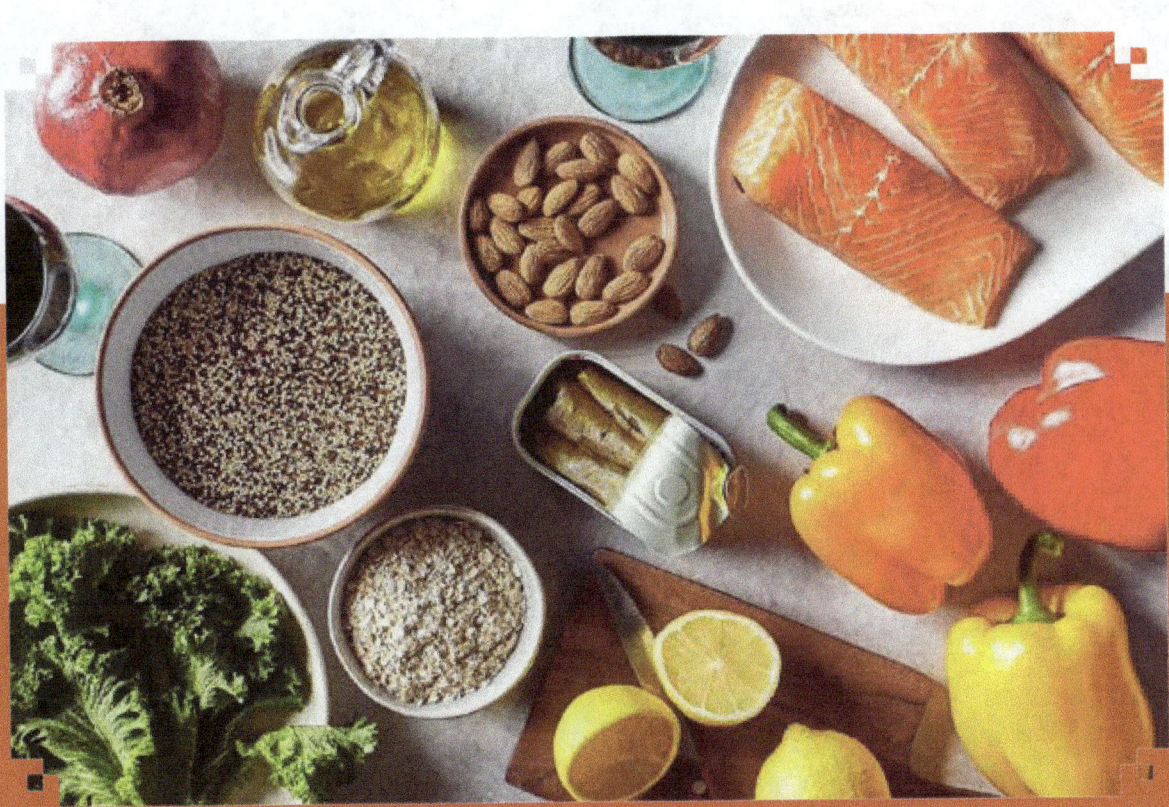

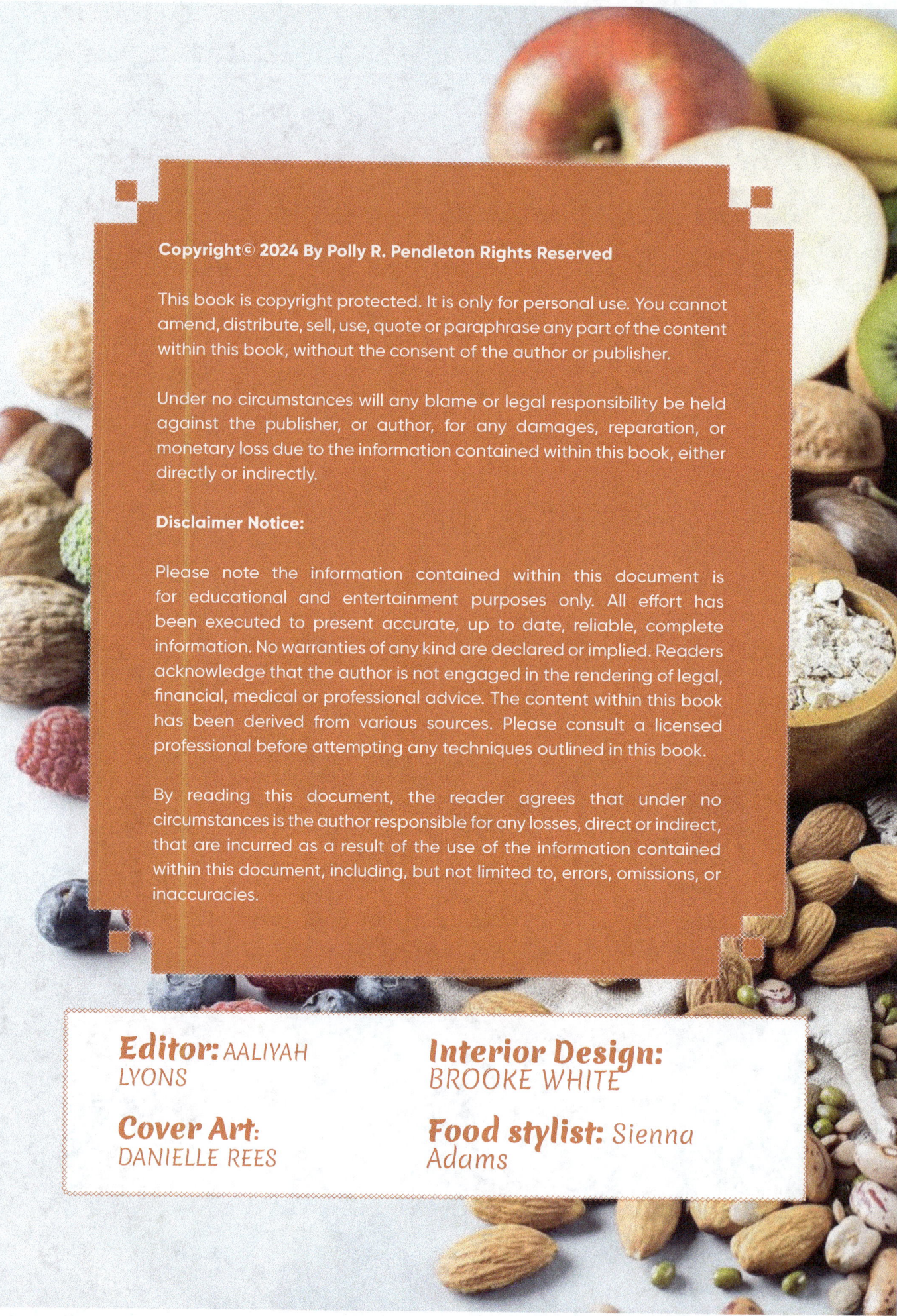

Editor: AALIYAH LYONS

Interior Design: BROOKE WHITE

Cover Art: DANIELLE REES

Food stylist: Sienna Adams

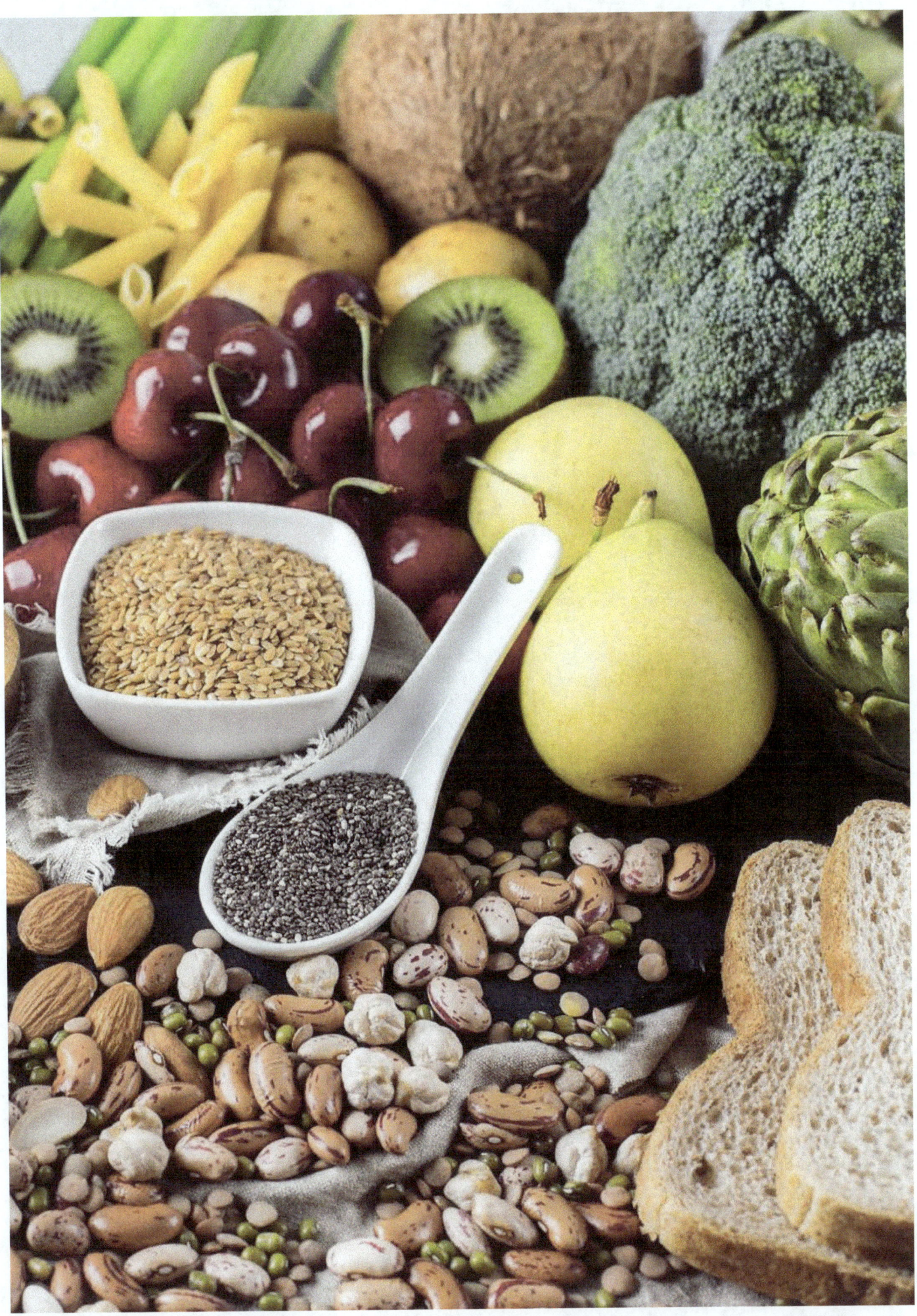

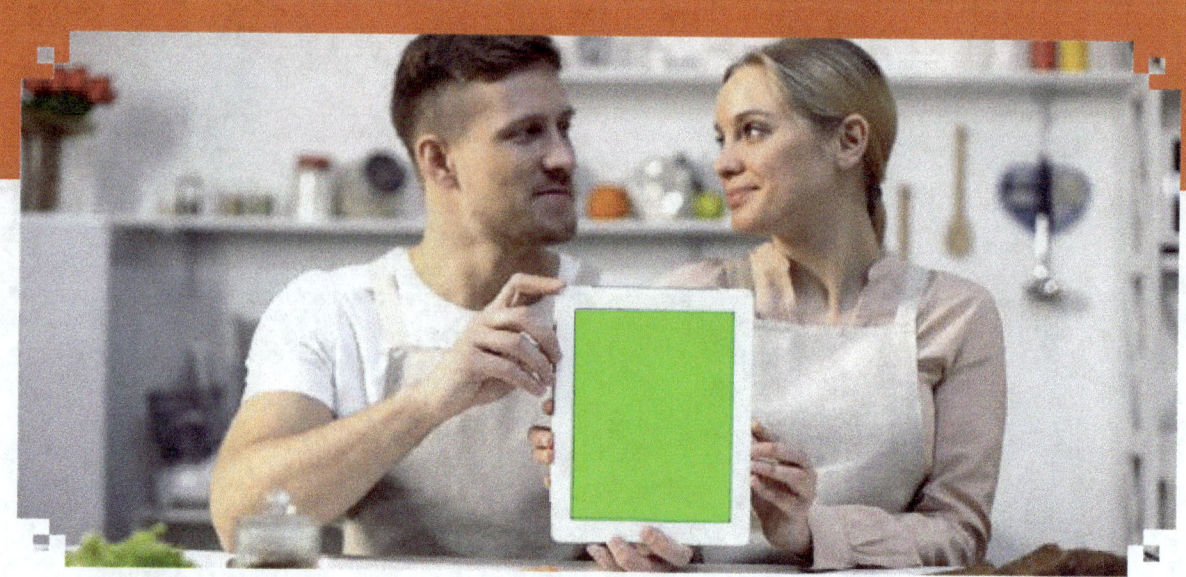

Table Of Contents

Introduction

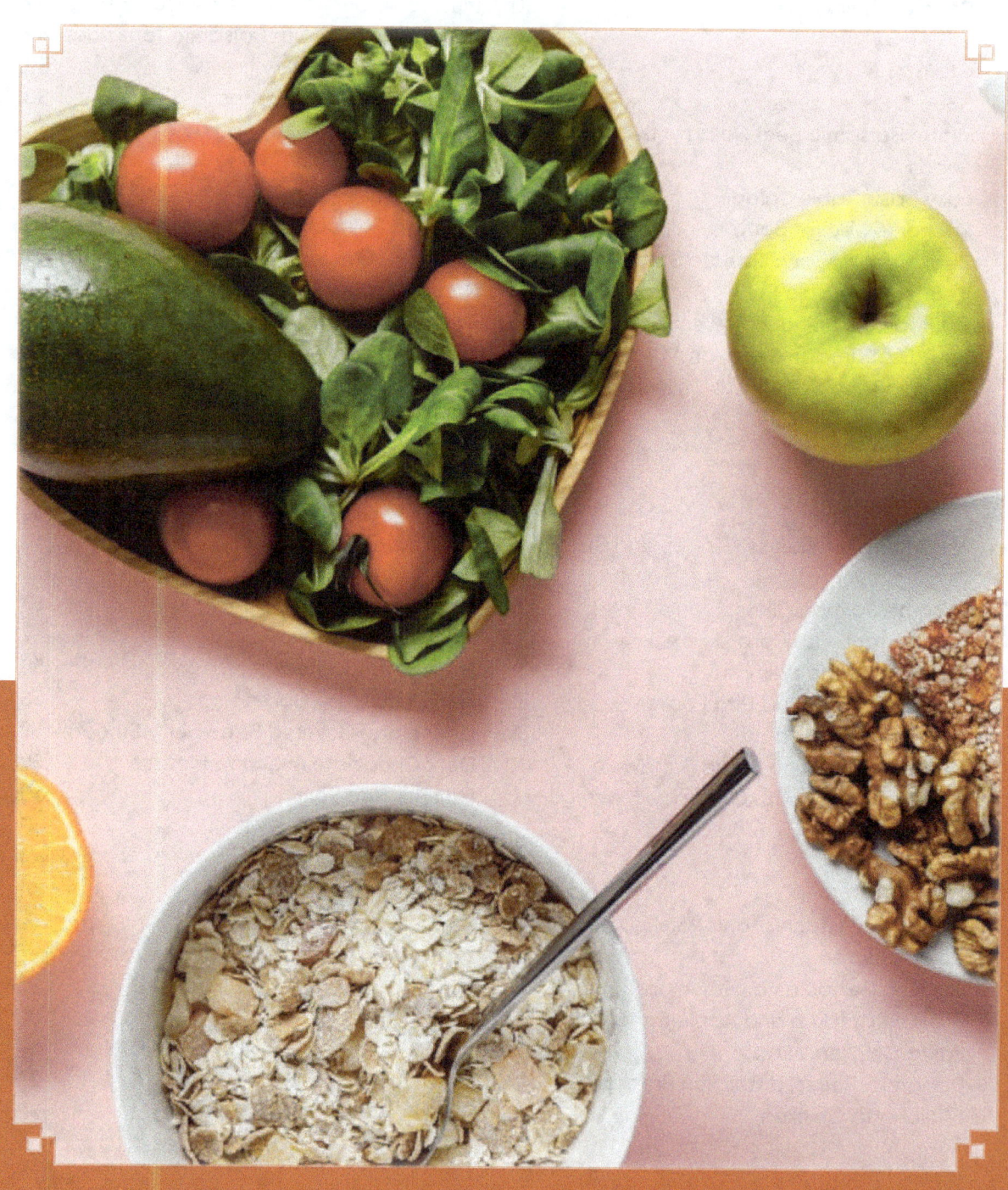

Prepare to embark on a culinary voyage that not only tantalizes your taste buds but also nourishes your heart and soul—and best of all, it's tailored for two. Within the pages of this cookbook lies a treasure trove of recipes meticulously curated to infuse your kitchen with flavor, vitality, and the essence of good health for you and your partner.

In a world inundated with fad diets and fast food temptations, the quest for heart-healthy sustenance often feels like a daunting challenge. But fear not, for you hold in your hands the blueprint for a delicious revolution—a revolution that proves you can savor every bite without compromising your well-being, and share it with someone you cherish.

Imagine the joy of sharing a meal with a loved one, knowing that each dish not only brings you closer together but also supports your journey toward optimal health, as a team. That's the beauty of the Heart Healthy Kitchen—a sanctuary where culinary creativity meets nutritional wisdom, and every meal is a celebration of life and vitality, enjoyed by both of you.

Within these pages, you'll discover a symphony of flavors inspired by cuisines from around the globe, perfectly portioned for two. From vibrant salads bursting with color to hearty stews brimming with wholesome goodness, each recipe is a testament to the artistry of healthy cooking and the pleasure of nourishing both body and soul.

But this cookbook is more than just a collection of recipes. It's a manifesto for a lifestyle rooted in wellness and enriched by the pleasures of the table, shared between two hearts. It's a reminder that the act of cooking is an expression of love, both for oneself and for those we hold dear, making every meal a gesture of care and connection.

So, as you embark on this culinary adventure together, may you find inspiration in every ingredient, joy in every preparation, and satisfaction in every bite. Here's to embracing the abundance of the Heart Healthy Kitchen and savoring the journey toward a happier, healthier "us".

Bon appétit!

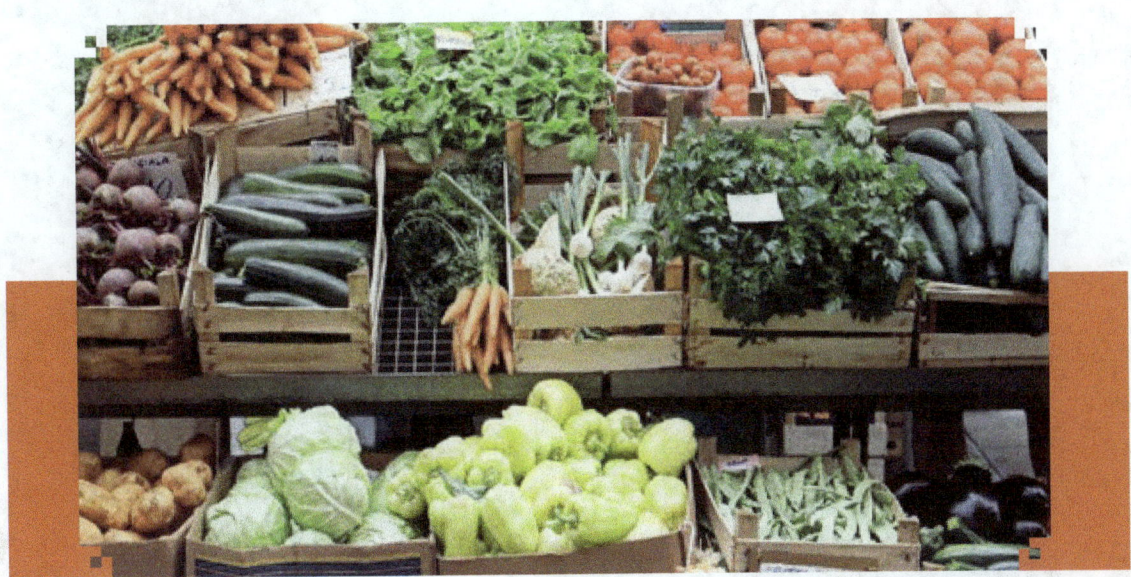

Chapter 1

Starting Your Heart-Healthy Journey

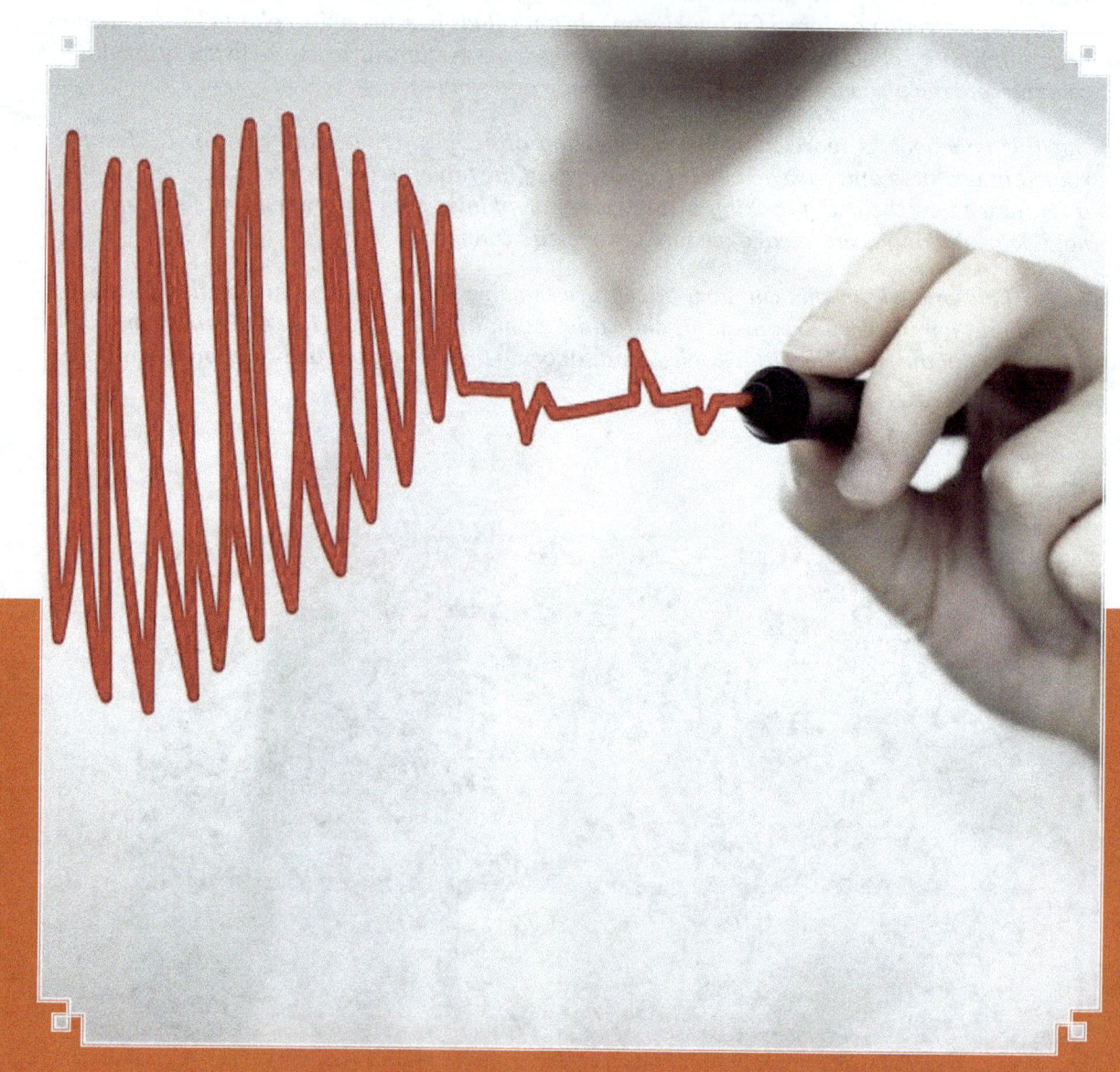

Exploring Heart Health Issues

Heart health stands as a cornerstone of overall well-being, with cardiovascular diseases being a leading cause of mortality worldwide. Understanding the complexities of heart health issues is essential for individuals seeking to protect themselves and their loved ones from such conditions.

Heart disease refers to a range of conditions that affect the heart, including coronary artery disease, heart rhythm disorders, heart valve defects, and congenital heart defects. These conditions can lead to various complications, such as heart attacks, heart failure, and strokes. Heart disease is often caused by a combination of factors, including genetics, lifestyle choices, and underlying medical conditions like hypertension, diabetes, and high cholesterol. Symptoms of heart disease may include chest pain, shortness of breath, fatigue, and irregular heartbeats. Early detection and management of risk factors are crucial in preventing the progression of heart disease and reducing the risk of complications.

A heart-healthy diet is a dietary approach that prioritizes foods known to support heart health and minimize the risk of cardiovascular disease. It typically emphasizes whole, nutrient-dense foods such as fruits, vegetables, whole grains, lean proteins, and healthy fats. These foods are rich in vitamins, minerals, antioxidants, and fiber, which can help regulate blood pressure, cholesterol levels, and inflammation in the body. A heart-healthy diet also limits the intake of processed foods, sugary beverages, trans fats, and excessive sodium, all of which are associated with an increased risk of heart disease. By adopting a heart-healthy diet and making lifestyle changes such as regular exercise and stress management, individuals can promote cardiovascular health and reduce their risk of heart disease.

• Advantages of a Heart-Friendly Diet

A heart-friendly diet offers numerous advantages, ranging from reducing the risk of cardiovascular diseases to enhancing overall health and vitality. Let's delve into some of the key benefits:

LOWER RISK OF HEART DISEASE

One of the most significant advantages of a heart-friendly diet is its ability to lower the risk of heart disease. By focusing on whole, nutrient-rich foods and minimizing processed and high-fat options, individuals can support their cardiovascular health. The inclusion of fruits, vegetables, whole grains, lean proteins, and healthy fats provides essential nutrients while helping to regulate blood pressure and cholesterol levels, key risk factors for heart disease.

IMPROVED HEART FUNCTION

A diet rich in heart-healthy foods can promote optimal heart function. Nutrient-dense foods such as fatty fish, nuts, seeds, and olive oil contain omega-3 fatty acids and monounsaturated fats, which have been shown to support heart health. These fats help reduce inflammation, lower triglyceride levels, and improve overall circulation, contributing to a healthier heart.

ENHANCED WEIGHT MANAGEMENT

Maintaining a healthy weight is crucial for heart health, and a heart-friendly diet can support weight management goals. By emphasizing whole foods that are low in calories and high in nutrients, individuals can feel satisfied while consuming fewer calories. Additionally, incorporating regular physical activity alongside a balanced diet can further support weight loss efforts and improve overall cardiovascular fitness.

REDUCED RISK OF CHRONIC DISEASES

In addition to lowering the risk of heart disease, a heart-friendly diet can also reduce the risk of other chronic diseases. The consumption of fruits, vegetables, whole grains, and lean proteins provides a wide array of vitamins, minerals, antioxidants, and fiber, which have been shown to have protective effects against conditions such as diabetes, cancer, and stroke.

INCREASED ENERGY AND VITALITY

Eating a diet rich in whole, nutrient-dense foods can boost energy levels and enhance overall vitality. By providing the body with the nutrients it needs to function optimally, a heart-friendly diet can help individuals feel more energetic, alert, and focused throughout the day. This increase in energy can also translate to improved performance during physical activity, further supporting heart health.

BETTER MOOD AND MENTAL HEALTH

There is growing evidence to suggest that diet plays a significant role in mental health and well-being. A heart-friendly diet that includes plenty of fruits, vegetables, whole grains, and healthy fats can support brain health and neurotransmitter function, which may contribute to improved mood and reduced risk of depression and anxiety.

Nourishing Your Heart with Food

The notion of "you are what you eat" couldn't be truer when it comes to heart health. Every morsel we consume has the potential to either nourish or harm our cardiovascular system. Understanding which foods can truly benefit our hearts is the first step towards adopting a heart-healthy lifestyle.

- Recommended Food Choices

FRUITS AND VEGETABLES

Incorporating a colorful array of fruits and vegetables into your diet provides essential vitamins, minerals, antioxidants, and dietary fiber. These nutrients help lower blood pressure, reduce inflammation, and improve overall heart health. Aim to fill half your plate with fruits and vegetables at every meal for maximum benefits.

WHOLE GRAINS

Whole grains such as oats, quinoa, brown rice, and whole wheat are rich in fiber, which helps lower cholesterol levels and reduce the risk of heart disease. Choose whole grain options over refined grains to provide your body with sustained energy and heart-healthy nutrients.

FATTY FISH

Fatty fish like salmon, mackerel, and sardines are excellent sources of omega-3 fatty acids, which are essential for heart health. Omega-3s help reduce inflammation, lower triglyceride levels, and decrease the risk of arrhythmias. Aim to include fatty fish in your diet at least twice a week for optimal heart benefits.

LEAN PROTEINS

Opt for lean protein sources such as skinless poultry, beans, lentils, tofu, and legumes instead of fatty cuts of meat. These protein sources are lower in saturated fat and cholesterol, making them heart-healthy choices that support muscle growth and repair.

Healthy Fats: Incorporating sources of healthy fats such as nuts, seeds, avocados, and olive oil into your diet can improve cholesterol levels and reduce the risk of heart disease. These fats are rich in monounsaturated and polyunsaturated fats, which help protect the heart and support overall health.

• Dietary Items to Limit or Exclude

TRANS FATS

Trans fats, often found in processed and fried foods, raise bad cholesterol levels (LDL) while lowering good cholesterol levels (HDL), increasing the risk of heart disease. Avoid foods containing partially hydrogenated oils and opt for healthier cooking methods such as baking, grilling, or steaming.

SATURATED FATS

While saturated fats are not entirely off-limits, they should be consumed in moderation. Limit intake of foods high in saturated fats such as red meat, full-fat dairy products, and butter. Instead, choose leaner cuts of meat and opt for low-fat or fat-free dairy options.

ADDED SUGARS AND SUGARY BEVER-AGES

Excess sugar consumption can lead to weight gain, inflammation, and an increased risk of heart disease. Minimize your intake of sugary snacks, desserts, and sugary beverages such as soda, fruit juices, and energy drinks. Instead, satisfy your sweet tooth with naturally sweetened fruits or opt for water, herbal tea, or sparkling water as refreshing alternatives.

EXCESSIVE SODIUM

High sodium intake can contribute to high blood pressure, a major risk factor for heart disease. Limit your consumption of processed foods, canned soups, salty snacks, and restaurant meals, which are often high in sodium. Instead, flavor your meals with herbs, spices, lemon juice, or vinegar to enhance taste without adding extra salt.

Perfecting the Art of Cooking for a Pair

Cooking for two presents a unique opportunity to create intimate dining experiences while efficiently managing portions and ingredients. Whether you're cooking for a romantic dinner or simply sharing a meal with a loved one, mastering the art of cooking for two can enhance both culinary skills and relationship dynamics.

• Efficient Grocery Shopping Strategies

Efficient grocery shopping is the cornerstone of successful meal preparation for couples. Here are some strategies to optimize your shopping experience and ensure you have everything you need for cooking for two:

• Plan Ahead: Before heading to the grocery store, take inventory of your pantry, fridge, and freezer, and create a meal plan for the week. This will help you identify which ingredients you already have and what items you need to purchase.
• Make a List: Compile a comprehensive shopping list based on your meal plan, including all the ingredients you'll need for each recipe. Organize your list by categories such as produce, dairy, proteins, and pantry staples to streamline your shopping trip.
• Stick to the List: While at the store, resist the temptation to deviate from your shopping list. Impulse purchases can lead to overspending and unnecessary food waste. Stay focused on purchasing

only the items you need for your planned meals.

- Buy in Bulk: When feasible, purchase non-perishable items such as grains, legumes, and spices in bulk to save money and reduce packaging waste. Consider investing in a membership to a warehouse club for additional savings on staple items.
- Utilize Technology: Take advantage of grocery shopping apps and online ordering services to streamline the shopping process. Many stores offer curbside pickup or home delivery options, saving you time and minimizing exposure to crowded stores.

- Expert Tips for Meal Planning

Meal planning is essential for efficient cooking for two. Follow these expert tips to streamline your meal planning process and ensure delicious and satisfying meals:

- Choose Versatile Ingredients: Select ingredients that can be used in multiple recipes to minimize waste and maximize versatility. For example, a rotisserie chicken can be repurposed into salads, sandwiches, soups, and pasta dishes throughout the week.
- Embrace Batch Cooking: Prepare larger quantities of certain foods, such as grains, proteins, and sauces, and portion them out for multiple meals. Batch cooking saves time and allows for easy assembly of meals throughout the week.
- Incorporate Leftovers: Plan meals that yield leftovers and incorporate them into subsequent meals. For example, leftover roasted vegetables can be added to salads, grain bowls, or omelets for a quick and nutritious meal.
- Keep It Simple: Focus on recipes that are easy to prepare with minimal ingredients

and cooking techniques. Simple dishes like stir-fries, sheet pan meals, and one-pot wonders are ideal for cooking for two and require less time and effort in the kitchen.
- Be Flexible: Remain flexible with your meal plan and adapt it based on changing schedules, preferences, and ingredient availability. Don't be afraid to swap ingredients or recipes as needed to accommodate your tastes and needs.

In the realm of heart-healthy diets tailored for two, there lies an abundance of potential for shared experiences, culinary exploration, and mutual growth. Cooking for oneself or with loved ones becomes an expression of self-care, nurturing, and commitment to a future of well-being. Through the art of creating heart-healthy meals, individuals fortify their bodies and create a foundation for a lifetime of shared joy, laughter, and contentment. In the kitchen and beyond, the heart-healthy diet becomes a symbol of self-love, resilience, and the pursuit of a vibrant life.

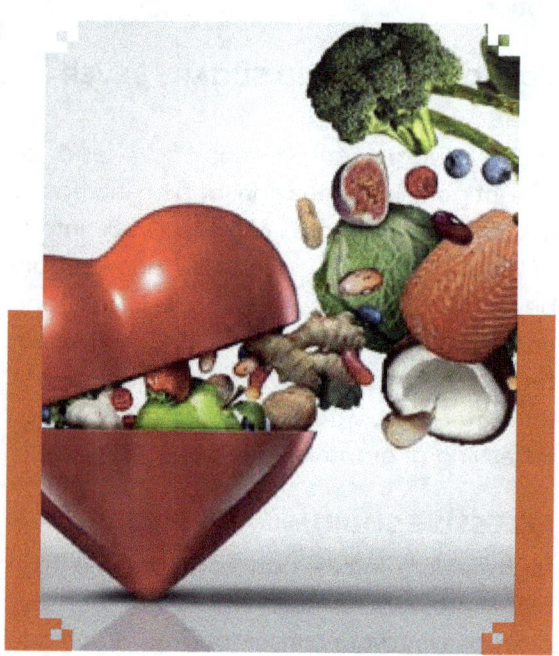

Chapter 2

4-Week Meal Plan

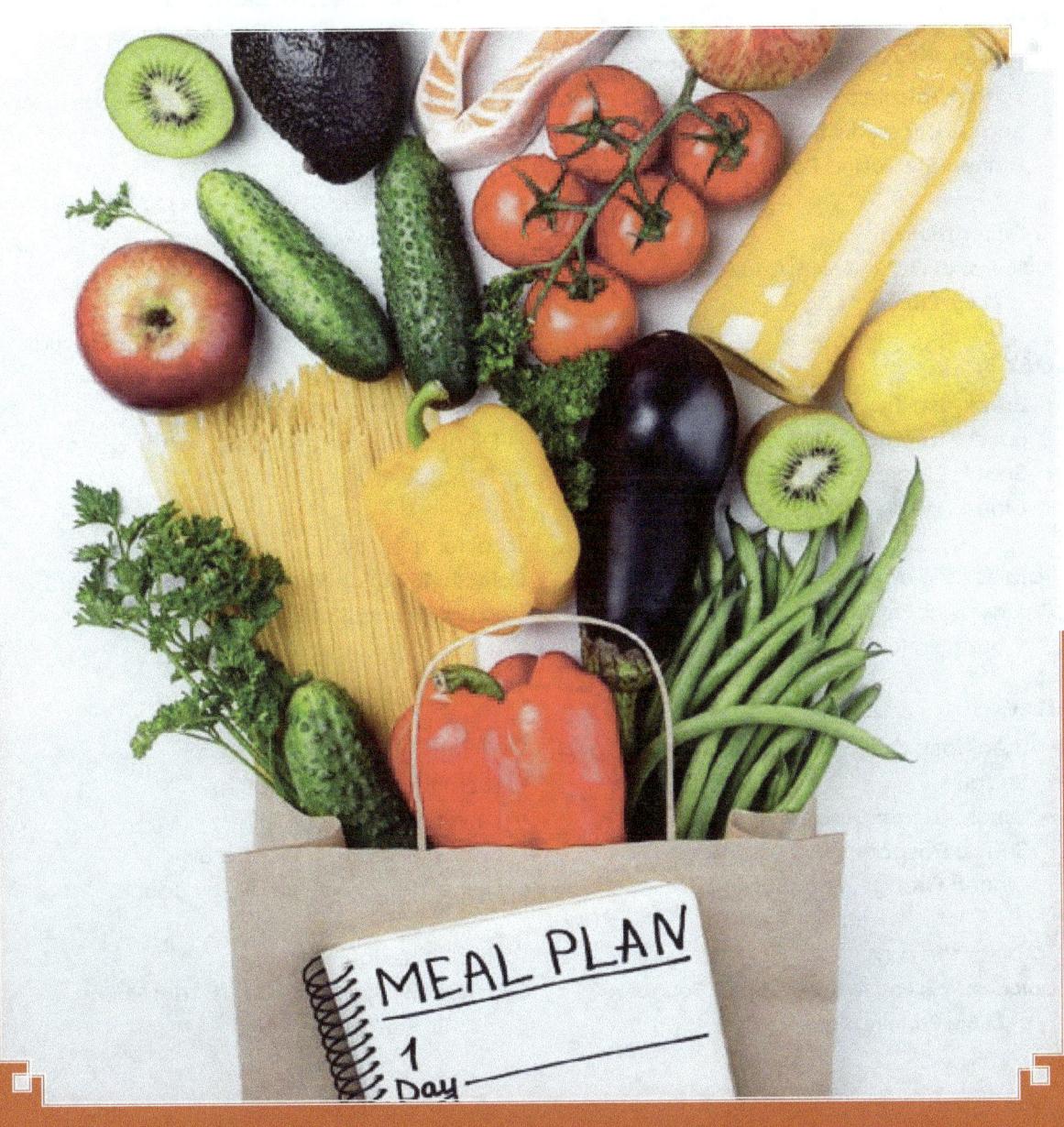

Week 1

DAY 1:
- Breakfast: Great Greens Smoothie Bowl
- Lunch: Crispy Trout with Herb
- Snack: Butter Crepes with a Hint of Citrus
- Dinner: Beef Stroganoff

Total for the day:
Calories: 1476; Fat: 76.96g; Carbs: 86.66g; Fiber: 9.8g; Protein: 108.49g

DAY 2:
- Breakfast: Orange and Oat Smoothie
- Lunch: Balsamic-Roasted Chicken Breasts
- Snack: Roasted Chickpeas
- Dinner: Steak and Potatoes

Total for the day:
Calories: 1043; Fat: 46.4g; Carbs: 88.1g; Fiber: 21.4g; Protein: 74.3g

DAY 3:
- Breakfast: Kiwi Clementine Smoothie
- Lunch: Tomato & Feta Salad
- Snack: Caprese Skewers
- Dinner: Herbed White Sea Bass

Total for the day:
Calories: 795; Fat: 46.4g; Carbs: 65.4g; Fiber: 14.2g; Protein: 60.8g

DAY 4:
- Breakfast: California Scrambled Eggs and Veggies
- Lunch: Ginger Sesame Salmon
- Snack: Raspberry-Lime Sorbet
- Dinner: Orange-Beef Stir-Fry

Total for the day:
Calories: 963; Fat: 49.5g; Carbs: 62.5g; Fiber: 22.5g; Protein: 61g

DAY 5:
- Breakfast: Classic French Toast
- Lunch: Mediterranean Tuna Wrap
- Snack: Black Bean Dip
- Dinner: Cilantro-Lime Brown Rice

Total for the day:
Calories: 486; Fat: 8.8g; Carbs: 65g; Fiber: 17g; Protein: 44g

DAY 6:
- Breakfast: Almost-Instant Oatmeal
- Lunch: Chicken and Quinoa Salad
- Snack: Zucchini Sticks
- Dinner: Chicken Pesto Pasta with Asparagus

Total for the day:
Calories: 1204; Fat: 57.9g; Carbs: 132.2g; Fiber: 13.8g; Protein: 68.9g

DAY 7:
- Breakfast: Greek Yogurt Topped with Almonds
- Lunch: Fresh Salmon Salad Pita Pocket
- Snack: Parsley Mushrooms
- Dinner: Beef Tenderloin with Balsamic Tomatoes

Total for the day:
Calories: 1079; Fat: 58.4g; Carbs: 63.6g; Fiber: 11g; Protein: 83.4g

Week 2

DAY 1:
- Breakfast: Omelet Waffles
- Lunch: Spicy Bean Chili
- Snack: Blueberry-Ricotta Swirl
- Dinner: Pork Loin with Figgy Sauce

Total for the day:
Calories: 969; Fat: 28.3g; Carbs: 111g; Fiber: 25.1g; Protein: 63g

DAY 2:

- Breakfast: Herb and Goat Cheese Egg White Omelet
- Lunch: Sprouted-Grain Pizza Toast
- Snack: Honey Ricotta with Espresso and Chocolate Chips
- Dinner: Mushroom and Red Wine Braised Beef

Total for the day:

Calories: 1287; Fat: 68.5g; Carbs: 77g; Fiber: 10g; Protein: 80g

DAY 3:

- Breakfast: Almond Butter and Blueberry Smoothie
- Lunch: Mint and Garlic Marinated Lamb Chops
- Snack: Garlicky Green Beans
- Dinner: Chicken & Veggie Parcel

Total for the day:

Calories: 1090; Fat: 67.6g; Carbs: 62.4g; Fiber: 23.4g; Protein: 73.7g

DAY 4:

- Breakfast: Classic French Toast
- Lunch: Chickpea Gyros
- Snack: Butternut Squash Fries
- Dinner: Steak with Red Onions, Peppers, and Mushrooms

Total for the day:

Calories: 702; Fat: 43.5g; Carbs: 77g; Fiber: 10.8g; Protein: 44.5g

DAY 5:

- Breakfast: Kiwi Clementine Smoothie
- Lunch: Caramelized Onions
- Snack: Honey Ricotta with Espresso and Chocolate Chips
- Dinner: Chicken and Broccoli Stir-Fry

Total for the day:

Calories: 649; Fat: 23.6g; Carbs: 82.1g; Fiber: 10.18g; Protein: 33.45g

DAY 6:

- Breakfast: Apricot-Orange Bread
- Lunch: Chicken & Broccoli Casserole
- Snack: Chia Seed Pudding
- Dinner: Haddock Tacos with Cabbage Slaw

Total for the day:

Calories: 885; Fat: 40.6g; Carbs: 66g; Fiber: 20.4g; Protein: 65.4g

DAY 7:

- Breakfast: Greek Yogurt Topped with Almonds
- Lunch: Roasted Eggplant Sandwiches
- Snack: Frozen Mango Treat
- Dinner: Lemon-Basil Chicken with Baby Bell Peppers

Total for the day:

Calories: 1315; Fat: 46.7g; Carbs: 148.9g; Fiber: 21.5g; Protein: 82.9g

Week 3

DAY 1:

- Breakfast: Orange and Oat Smoothie
- Lunch: Bruschetta Chicken
- Snack: Black Bean Dip
- Dinner: Open-Faced Lemon Pepper Tuna Melt

Total for the day:

Calories: 842; Fat: 40.1g; Carbs: 72g; Fiber: 16.2g; Protein: 55.2g

DAY 2:

- Breakfast: Classic French Toast
- Lunch: Black Bean and Red Pepper Stuffed Zucchini
- Snack: Parsley Mushrooms
- Dinner: Sesame Salmon Fillets

Total for the day:

Calories: 884; Fat: 47g; Carbs: 61.2g; Fiber: 19g; Protein: 62.6g

DAY 3:
- Breakfast: Great Greens Smoothie Bowl
- Lunch: Sautéed Spinach with Pumpkin Seeds
- Snack: Honey Ricotta with Espresso and Chocolate Chips
- Dinner: Toasted Chicken and Apple Sandwich

Total for the day:

Calories: 1065; Fat: 45.1g; Carbs: 117g; Fiber: 16.9g; Protein: 58.4g

DAY 4:
- Breakfast: Avocado and Tomato Toasts
- Lunch: Cauliflower Steak with Arugula-Basil Pesto
- Snack: Cherry-Vanilla Cupcake
- Dinner: Apple-Cinnamon Baked Pork Chops

Total for the day:

Calories: 1101; Fat: 61g; Carbs: 94g; Fiber: 24g; Protein: 54g

DAY 5:
- Breakfast: Omelet Waffles
- Lunch: Easy Basic Table Salad
- Snack: Caprese Skewers
- Dinner: Avocado and Tuna Salad Sandwich

Total for the day:

Calories: 1704; Fat: 112.5g; Carbs: 118.4g; Fiber: 16g; Protein: 72.8g

DAY 6:
- Breakfast: Herb and Goat Cheese Egg White Omelet
- Lunch: Warm Balsamic Beet Salad with Sunflower Seeds
- Snack: Fresh Berry Parfait
- Dinner: Haddock Tacos with Cabbage Slaw

Total for the day:

Calories: 851; Fat: 32.5g; Carbs: 82g; Fiber: 19g; Protein: 60g

DAY 7:
- Breakfast: Almost-Instant Oatmeal
- Lunch: Quinoa and Spinach Power Salad
- Snack: Garlicky Green Beans
- Dinner: Mushroom and Red Wine Braised Beef

Total for the day:

Calories: 1333; Fat: 61.9g; Carbs: 129.5g; Fiber: 26.2g; Protein: 75.9g

Week 4

DAY 1:
- Breakfast: California Scrambled Eggs and Veggies
- Lunch: Grilled Garlic Rosemary Pork Tenderloin
- Snack: Butter Crepes with a Hint of Citrus
- Dinner: South Asian Baked Salmon

Total for the day:

Calories: 954; Fat: 56g; Carbs: 40g; Fiber: 9.2g; Protein: 81g

DAY 2:
- Breakfast: Almond Butter and Blueberry Smoothie
- Lunch: Whole Branzino
- Snack: Stuffed Sweet Potatoes with Pistachios
- Dinner: Blueberry, Pistachio, and Parsley Chicken

Total for the day:

Calories: 1163; Fat: 51g; Carbs: 92g; Fiber: 22g; Protein: 96g

DAY 3:
- Breakfast: Apricot-Orange Bread

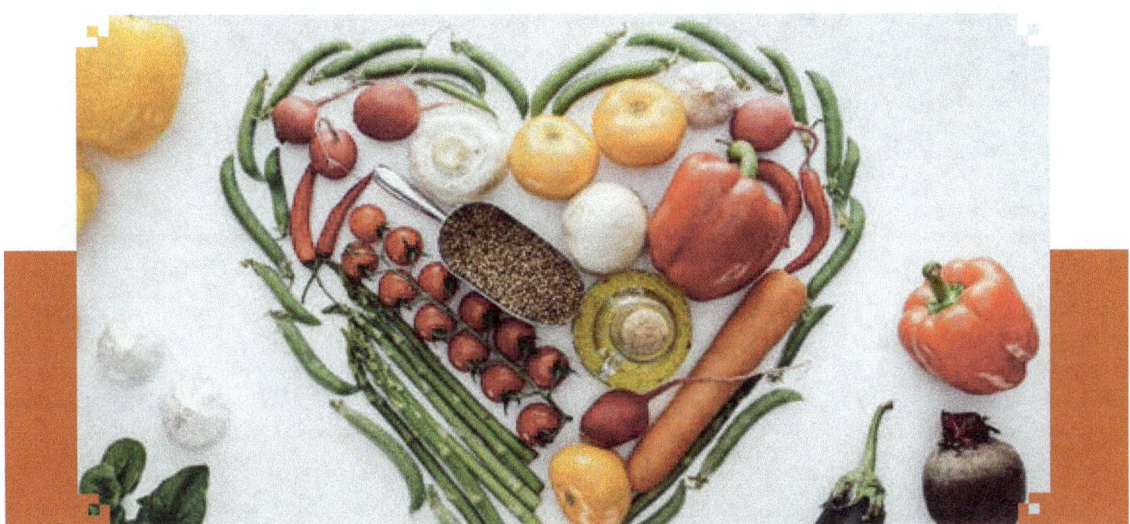

- Lunch: Tomato & Feta Salad
- Snack: Roasted Chickpeas
- Dinner: Mediterranean Tuna Wrap

Total for the day:
Calories: 658; Fat: 14.8g; Carbs: 94.3g; Fiber: 28.8g; Protein: 50.4g

DAY 4:
- Breakfast: Kiwi Clementine Smoothie
- Lunch: Mahi Mahi with Leeks, Ginger, and Baby Bok Choy
- Snack: Zucchini Sticks
- Dinner: Fajita Chicken Wraps

Total for the day:
Calories: 748; Fat: 31.6g; Carbs: 66.8g; Fiber: 13.1g; Protein: 74.9g

DAY 5:
- Breakfast: Omelet Waffles
- Lunch: Basil Tomato Crostini
- Snack: Cashew Cream Mousse
- Dinner: Orange-Beef Stir-Fry

Total for the day:

Calories: 901; Fat: 34.5g; Carbs: 89g; Fiber: 9.4g; Protein: 48g

DAY 6:
- Breakfast: Classic French Toast
- Lunch: Crispy Trout with Herb
- Snack: Black Bean Dip
- Dinner: Lemon Herb Beef Kabobs

Total for the day:
Calories: 1273; Fat: 71.96g; Carbs: 35.66g; Fiber: 8g; Protein: 120.49g

DAY 7:
- Breakfast: Almond Butter and Blueberry Smoothie
- Lunch: Sprouted-Grain Pizza Toast
- Snack: Stuffed Sweet Potatoes with Pistachios
- Dinner: Beef Stroganoff

Total for the day:
Calories: 1604; Fat: 92g; Carbs: 143g; Fiber: 29.3g; Protein: 66g

Chapter 3

Seasonings Delights

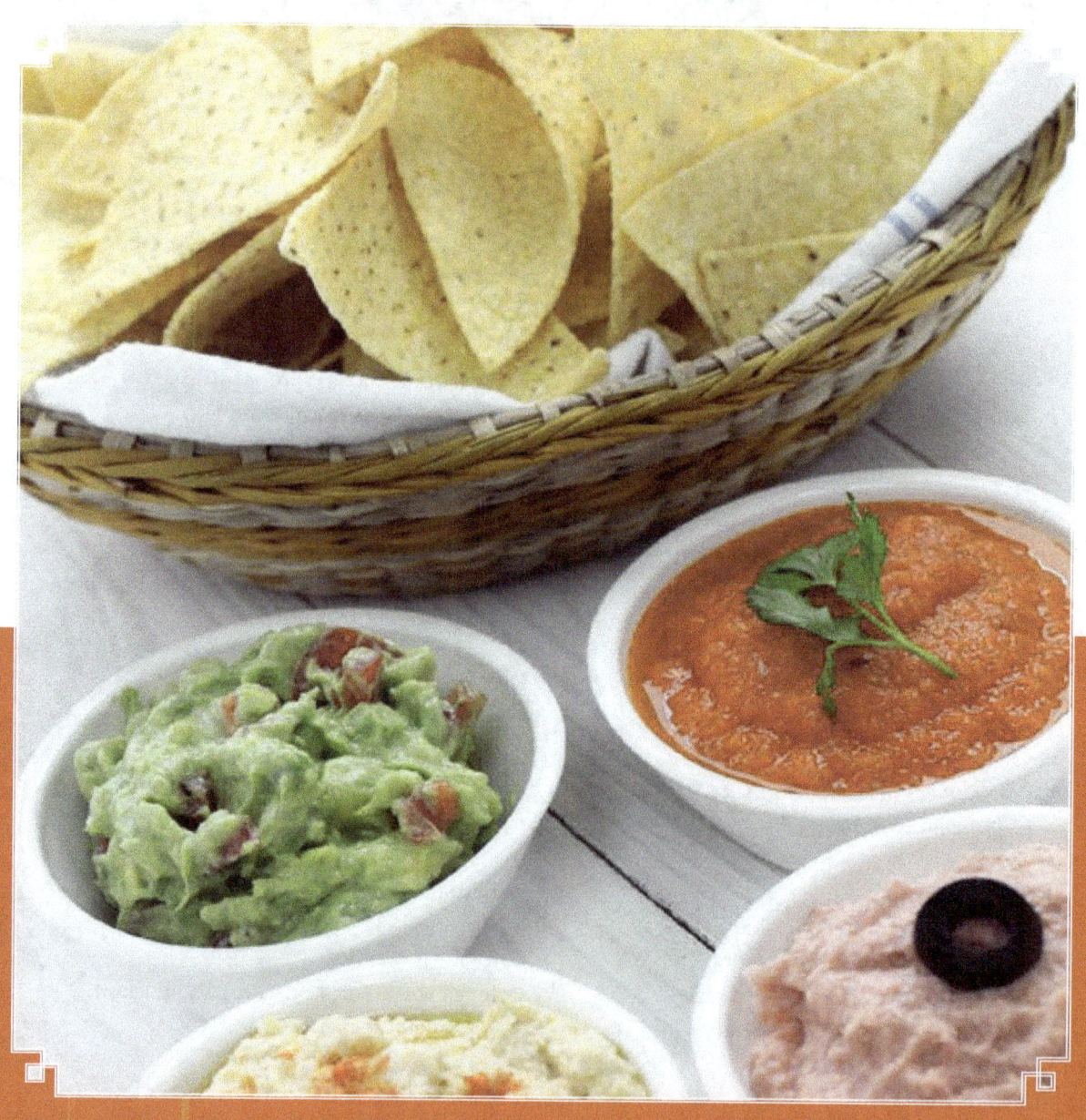

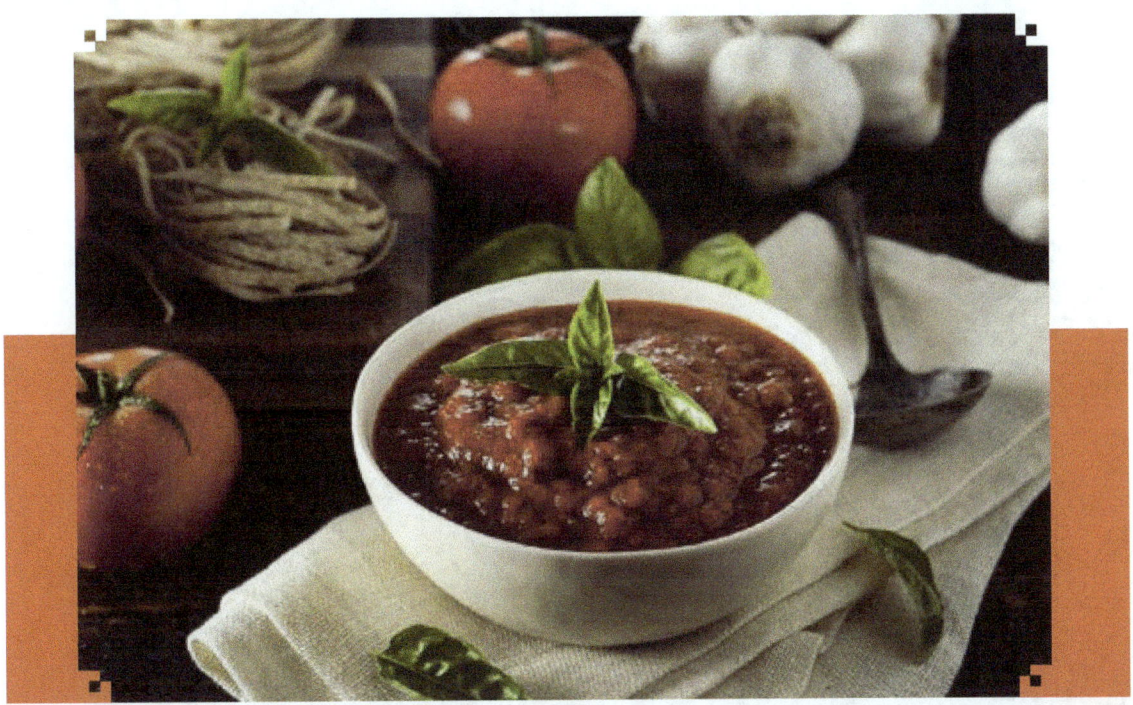

Balsamic Vinaigrette Dressing

Prep time: 5 minutes | Cook time: none | Serves 2

- ¼ cup balsamic vinegar
- 1 tablespoons extra virgin olive oil
- ½ tablespoon Dijon mustard
- ½ clove garlic, minced
- Salt and pepper to taste

1. In a small bowl, whisk together balsamic vinegar, olive oil, Dijon mustard, minced garlic, salt, and pepper.
2. Serve immediately or refrigerate for up to one week.

PER SERVING

Calories: 70 | Total Fat: 7g | Carbs: 2g | Fiber: 0g | Protein: 0g

Zesty Tomato Dressing

Prep time: 10 minutes | Cook time: none | Serves 2

- 1 cup no-salt-added tomato juice
- 2 medium green onions, thinly sliced
- 2 tablespoons fresh lemon juice
- 2 tablespoons red wine vinegar
- 1 teaspoon dried parsley, crumbled
- ¼ teaspoon pepper

1. In a medium glass bowl, whisk together the ingredients until the sugar is dissolved.
2. Cover and refrigerate for up to three days.

PER SERVING

Calories: 10 | Total Fat: 0.0 g |Carbs: 2 g | Fiber: 0 g | Protein: 0 g

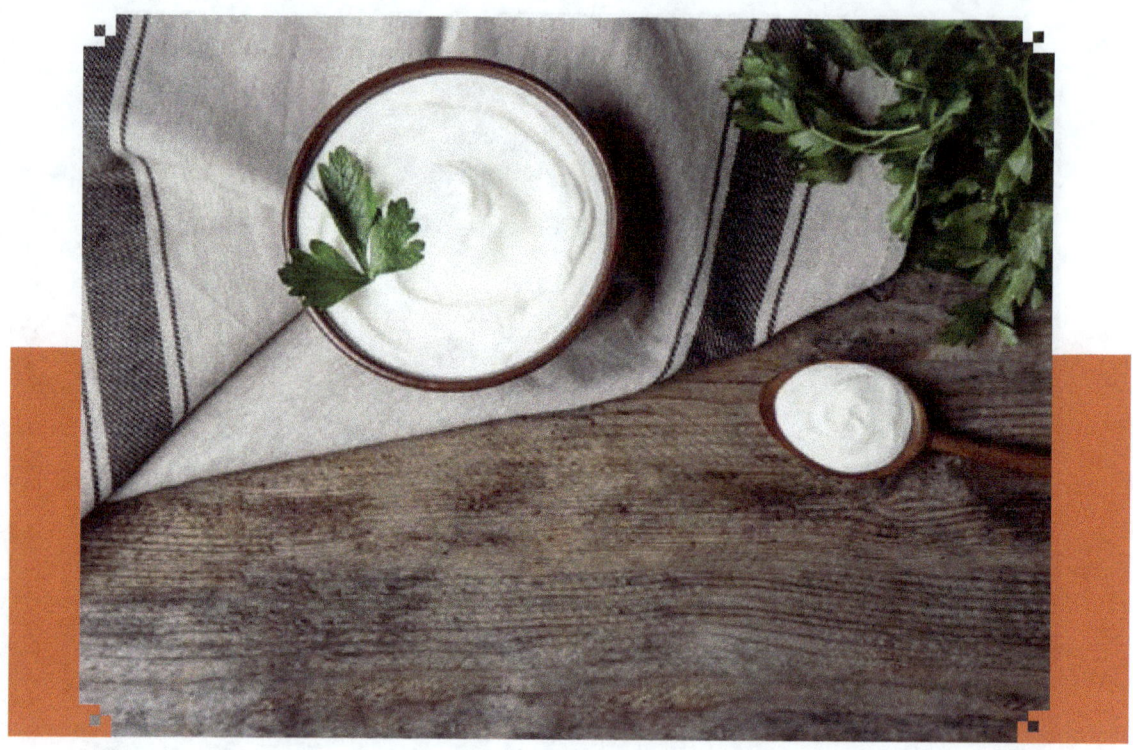

Honey Mustard Dip

Prep time: 5 minutes | Cook time: none | Serves 2

- ¼ cup Dijon mustard
- ¼ tablespoon honey
- ¼ tablespoon plain Greek yogurt
- ½ tablespoon lemon juice
- Salt and pepper to taste

1. In a small bowl, whisk together Dijon mustard, honey, Greek yogurt, lemon juice, salt, and pepper until smooth.
2. Adjust seasoning to taste.
3. Serve immediately or refrigerate for up to one week.

PER SERVING

Calories: 30 | Total Fat: 0g | Carbs: 7g | Fiber: 0g | Protein: 1g

Greek Yogurt Ranch Dip

Prep time: 5 minutes | Cook time: none | Serves 2

- ¼ cup plain Greek yogurt
- ½ tablespoon lemon juice
- ½ teaspoon dried dill
- ½ teaspoon dried parsley
- Salt and pepper to taste

1. In a mixing bowl, combine Greek yogurt, lemon juice, dried dill, dried parsley, garlic powder, salt, and pepper.
2. Stir until well combined.
3. Serve immediately or refrigerate for up to one week.

PER SERVING

Calories: 30 | Total Fat: 0g | Carbs: 2g | Fiber: 0g | Protein: 6g

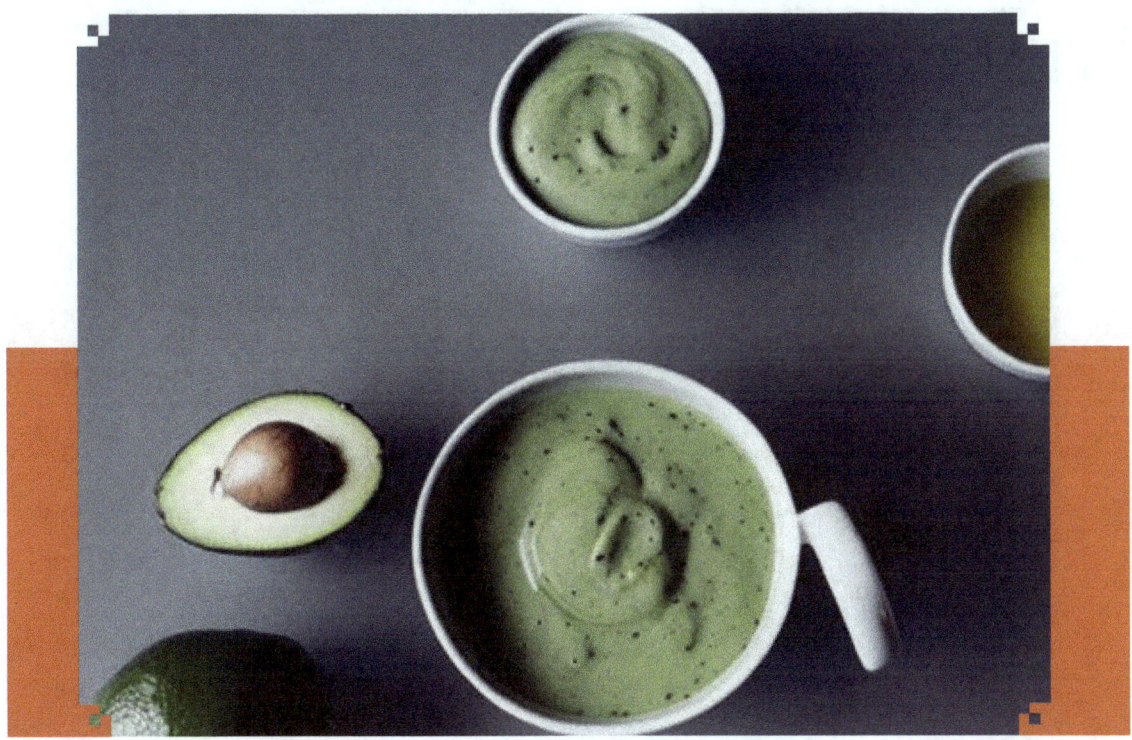

Honey Mustard Sauce

Prep time: 5 minutes | Cook time: none | Serves 2

- 2 tablespoons Dijon mustard
- 1 tablespoon honey
- 1 tablespoon apple cider vinegar
- Salt and pepper to taste

1. In a small bowl, whisk together the Dijon mustard, honey, apple cider vinegar, and olive oil until well combined.
2. Season with salt and pepper to taste.
3. Serve immediately or store in an airtight container in the refrigerator for up to 1 week.

PER SERVING

Calories: 85|Fat: 6g|Carbs: 8g|Fiber: 0g|Protein: 0g

Avocado Lime Dressing

Prep time: 5 minutes | Cook time: none | Serves 2

- ½ ripe avocado, peeled and pitted
- Juice of 2 limes
- 1 tablespoon extra virgin olive oil
- ½ tablespoon honey
- Salt and pepper to taste

1. In a blender or food processor, combine avocado, lime juice, olive oil, honey, salt, and pepper.
2. Blend until smooth and creamy.
3. Serve immediately or refrigerate for up to three days.

PER SERVING

Calories: 120 | Fat: 10g | Carbs: 8g | Fiber: 4g | Protein: 1g

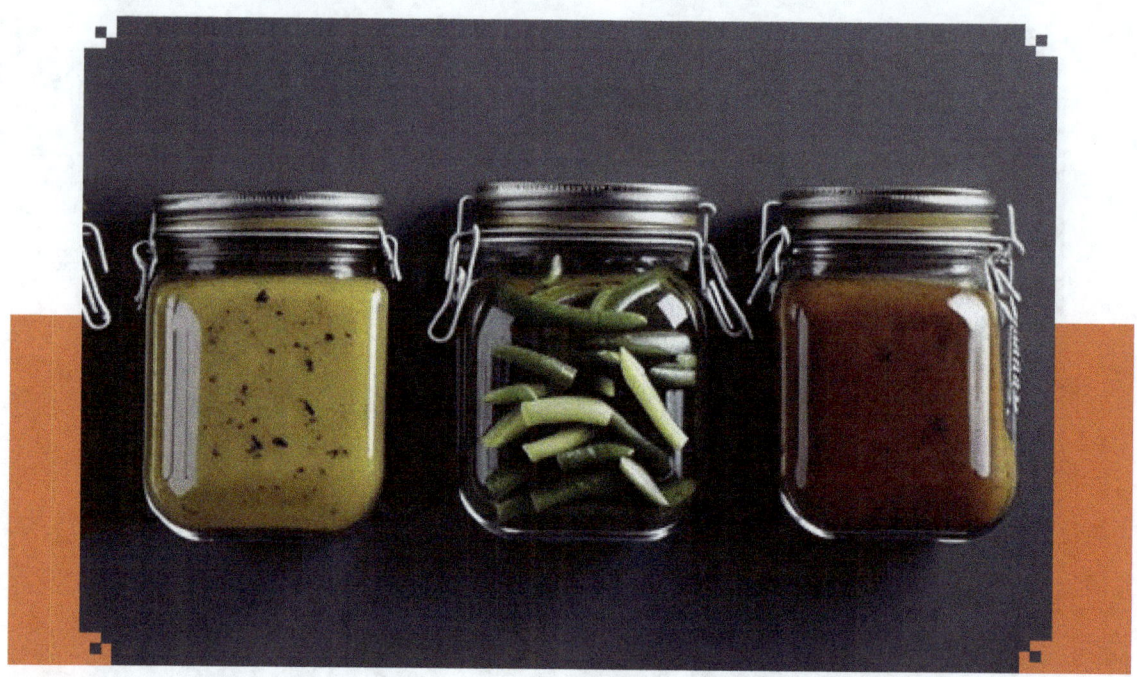

Simple Tomato Sauce

Prep time: 10 minutes | Cook time: 20 minutes |
Serves 2

- ¼ cup extra-virgin olive oil
- 3 garlic cloves, minced
- 2 pints grape tomatoes, halved
- 2 tablespoons chopped fresh basil
- ¼ teaspoon salt
- ¼ teaspoon freshly ground black pepper
- ¼ teaspoon red pepper flakes (optional)

1. In a large skillet, heat the oil over medium heat. until the tomatoes are softened and the sauce has thickened slightly.
2. Stir in the red pepper flakes (if using). ounces or more.

PER SERVING

Calories: 153 | Fat: 14g | Carbs: 15g | Fiber: 2g
| Protein: 2g

Chili Lime Marinade

Prep time: 10 minutes | Cook time: 5 minutes |
Serves 2

- ¼ cup canola oil
- zest and juice of 1 lime
- 2 tablespoons apple cider vinegar
- 1 tablespoon chili powder
- 1 teaspoon garlic powder
- 1 teaspoon onion powder
- ¼ teaspoon kosher or sea salt
- ¼ teaspoon ground black pepper

1. Whisk all the ingredients together, and store in an airtight container in the refrigerator for up to 5 days or freeze it for up to 2 months.

PER SERVING:

Calories: 266 | Fat: 27g | Carbs: 4g | Fiber: 1g
| Protein: 1g

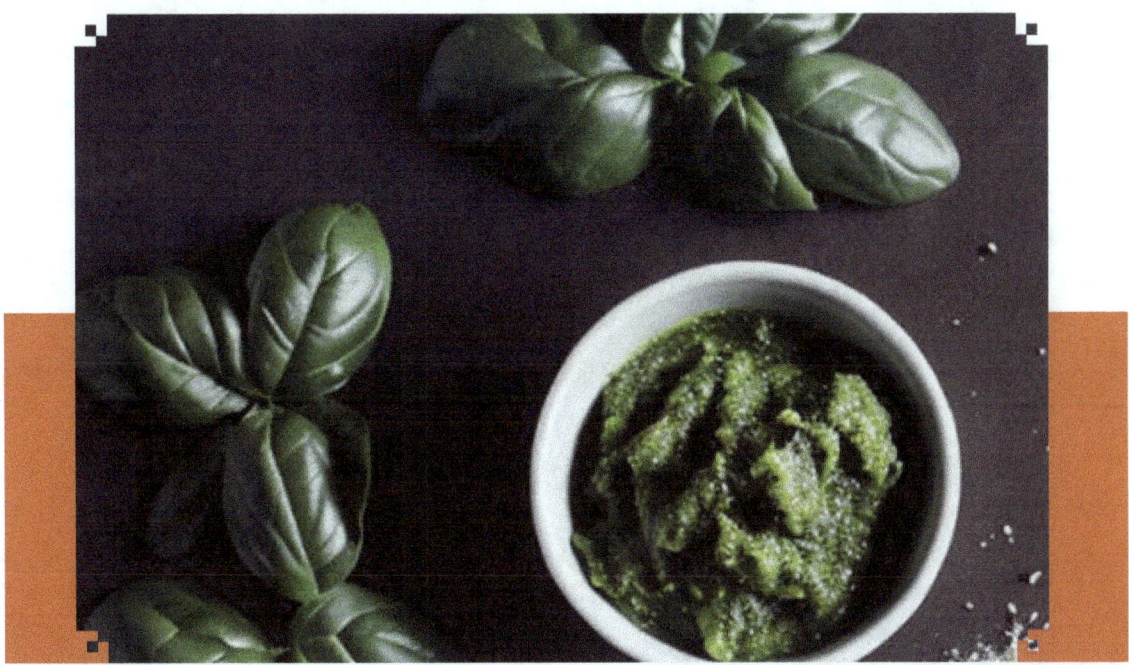

Tahini Yogurt Dressing

Prep time: 5 minutes | Cook time: none | Serves 2

- ¼ cup tahini
- ¼ cup plain Greek yogurt
- ½ tablespoon lemon juice
- ½ tablespoon water
- ½ clove garlic, minced
- Salt and pepper to taste

1. In a small bowl, whisk together tahini, Greek yogurt, lemon juice, water, minced garlic, salt, and pepper.
2. Adjust consistency with more water if needed.
3. Serve immediately or refrigerate for up to one week.

PER SERVING

Calories: 90 | Total Fat: 7g | Carbs: 4g | Fiber: 1g | Protein: 4g

Fresh Basil Pesto

Prep time: 10 minutes | Cook time: 5 minutes | Serves 2

- 2 cups fresh basil leaves, packed
- 1/4 cup grated Parmesan cheese
- 2 tablespoons pine nuts or walnuts
- 1/4 cup olive oil
- Salt and pepper to taste

1. In a food processor, combine the basil leaves, Parmesan cheese, pine nuts or walnuts, and minced garlic.
2. Pulse until finely chopped.
3. Serve immediately or store in an airtight container in the refrigerator for up to 1 week.

PER SERVING:

Calories: 250|Fat: 26g| Carbs: 2g| Fiber: 1g| Protein: 3g

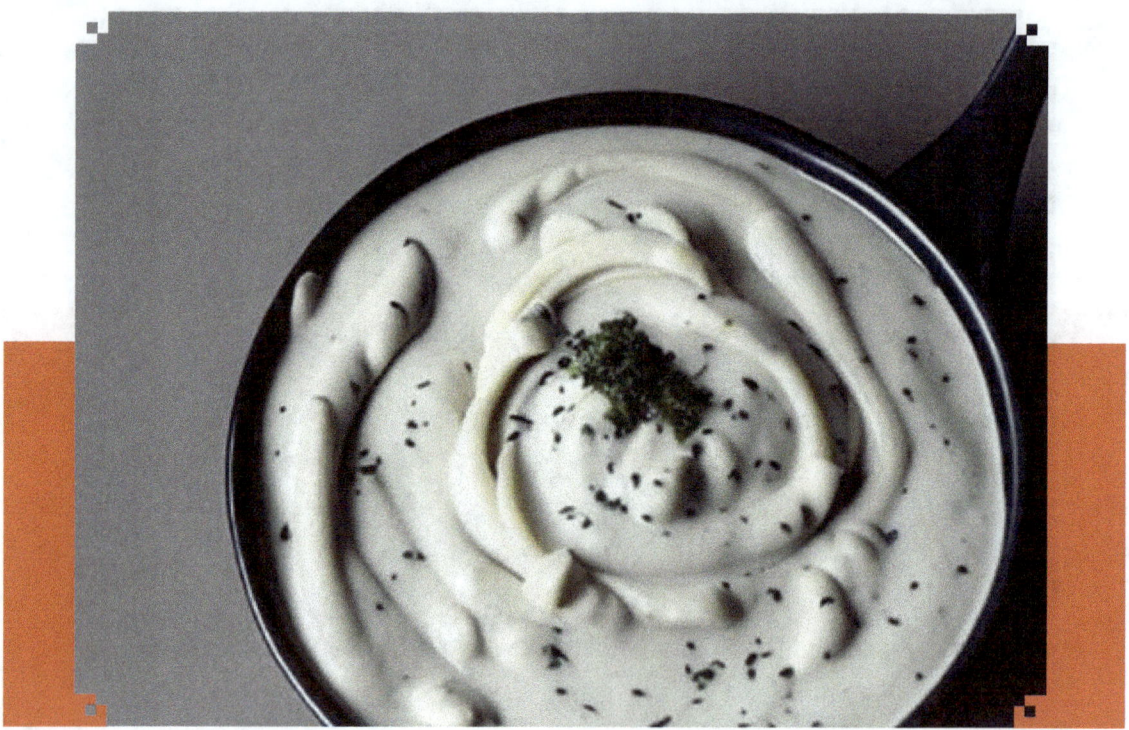

Creamy Avocado Dressing

Prep time: 5 minutes | Cook time: 3 minutes | Serves 2

- 1 ripe avocado, peeled and pitted
- 1/4 cup plain Greek yogurt
- 2 tablespoons fresh cilantro, chopped
- 1 tablespoon lime juice
- Salt and pepper to taste
- Water (optional, for desired consistency)

1. In a blender or food processor, combine the avocado, Greek yogurt, cilantro, lime juice, and minced garlic.
2. Season with salt and pepper to taste.

PER SERVING

Calories: 90 | Fat: 7g | Carbs: 6g | Fiber: 4g | Protein: 3g

Mustard and Green Onion Sauce

Prep time: 10 minutes | Cook time: none | Serves 2

- ½ cup light mayonnaise
- ½ cup fat-free plain Greek yogurt
- 2 tablespoons Dijon mustard (lowest sodium available)
- 3 tablespoons minced green onion
- ⅛ teaspoon garlic powder

1. In a medium bowl, whisk together all the ingredients.
2. Cover and refrigerate.

PER SERVING

Calories: 20 | Fat: 1.5 g |Carbs: 1 g | Fiber: 0 g | Protein: 1 g

Chapter 4

Breakfast Bonanza

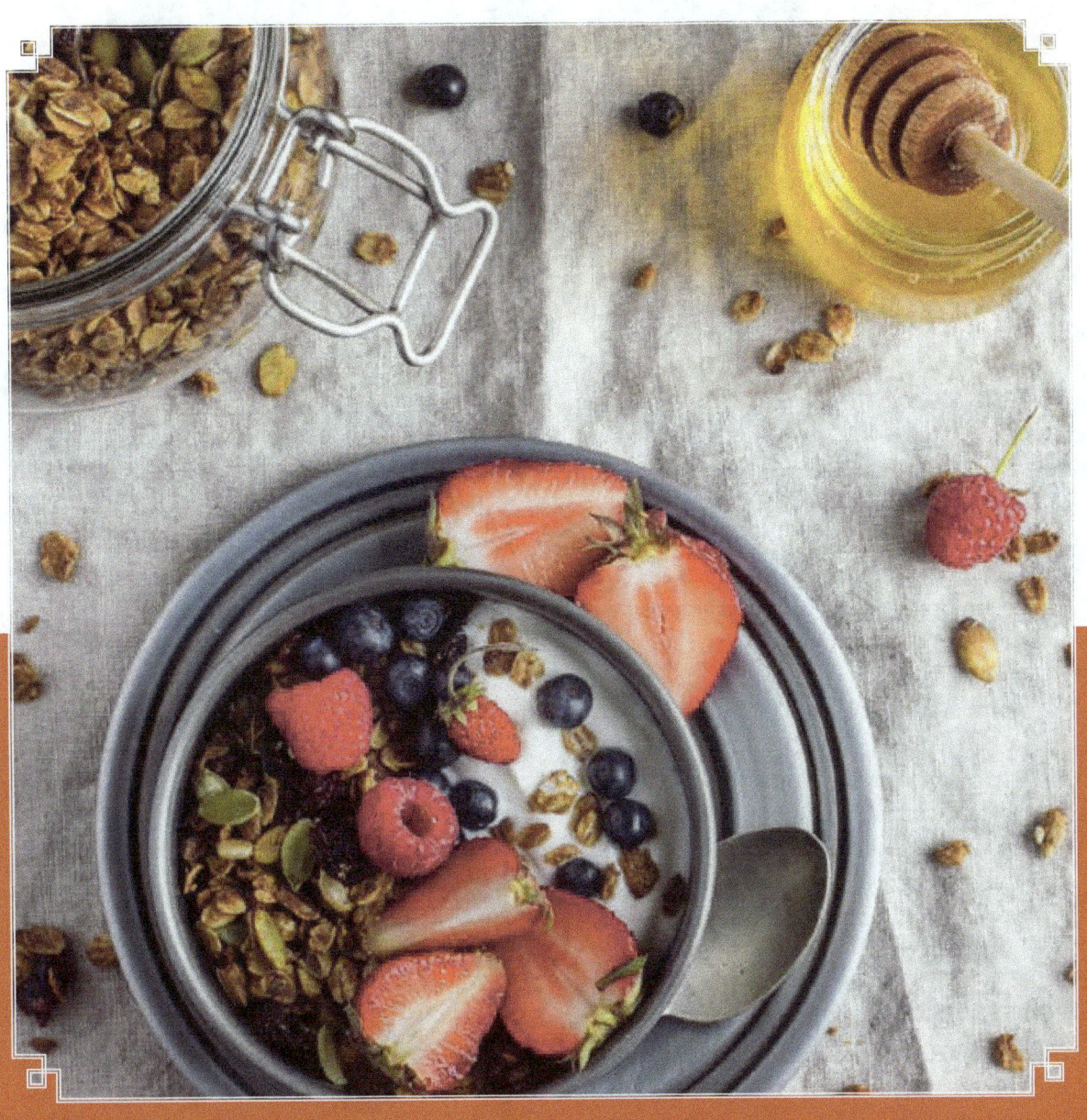

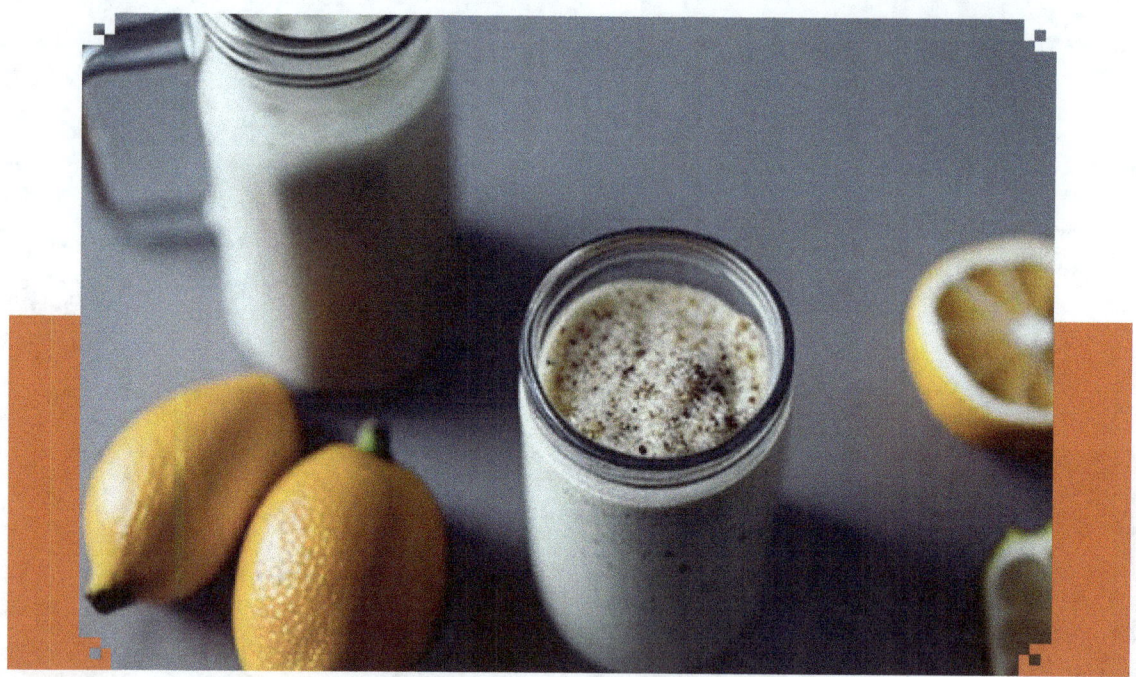

Great Greens Smoothie Bowl

Prep time: 10 minutes | Cook time: 3 minutes | Serves 2

- ¼ cup unsweetened coconut flakes
- 1 green apple, thinly sliced, divided
- 1 banana, cut into chunks
- 1 cup 1% milk
- ½ lemon, thinly sliced

1. In a small dry skillet, toast the coconut flakes over medium heat for 2 to 3 minutes, or until lightly browned. Set side.
2. For each serving, pour half the smoothie apple slices, half the lemon slices, and coconut flakes.

PER SERVING

Calories: 262 | Fat: 6.5g | Carbs: 47g | Fiber: 7.5g | Protein: 8g

Orange and Oat Smoothie

Prep time: 5 minutes | Cook time: none | Serves 2

- ½ cup rolled oats
- ½ banana, peeled and sliced
- 1¼ cups unsweetened almond milk
- 1 orange, peeled, sectioned and seeded
- ½ cup ice cubes

1. Add rolled oats in a high-speed blender and pulse until they are completely chopped.
2. Add in banana slices, almond milk and orange. Pulse to form a smooth mixture.
3. Pour in two serving glasses and add ice cubes in them.
4. Serve and enjoy!

PER SERVING

Calories: 202 | Fat: 6.4g | Carbs: 34.1g | Fiber: 6.4g | Protein: 5.3g

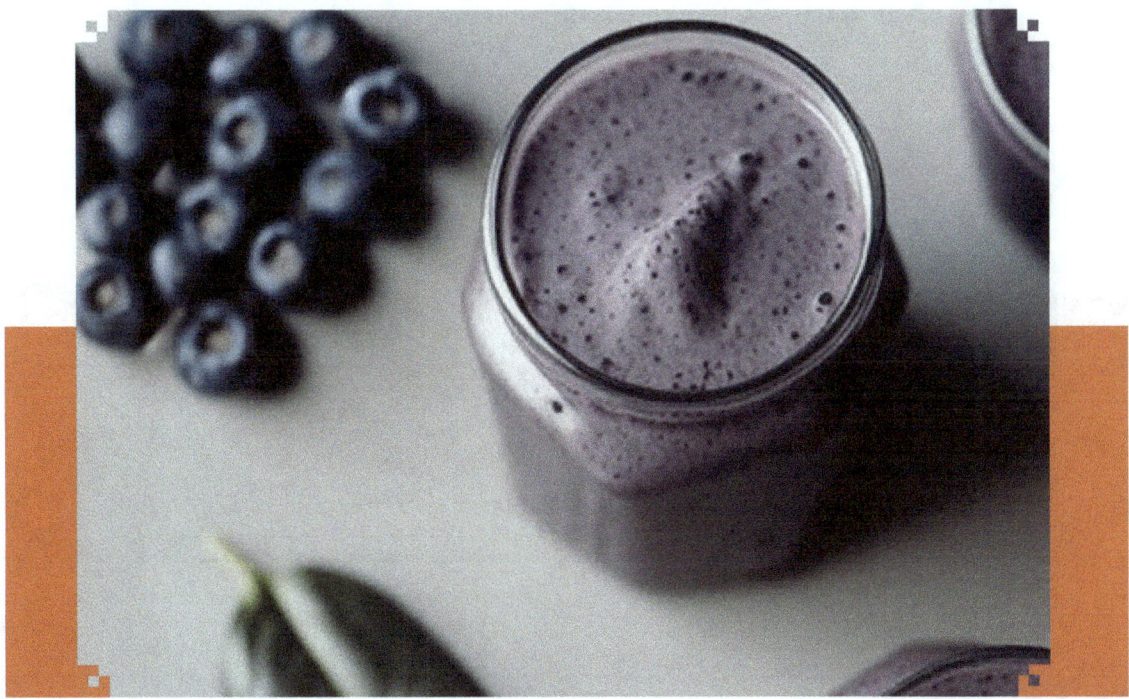

Apricot-Orange Bread

Prep time: 8 minutes | Cook time: 65 minutes |
Serves 2

- 1 package (6 oz) dried apricots, cut into small pieces
- 1 cup sugar
- 2 tbsp margarine
- ½ cup orange juice
- ½ cup pecans, chopped

1. Preheat oven to 350°F. Lightly oil two, 9- by 5-inch loaf pans.
2. Turn batter into prepared pans.
3. Cool for 5 minutes in pans. Remove rack before slicing.

PER SERVING:

Calories: 97| Fat: 2g| Fiber: 1g| Protein: 2g| Carbs: 18g

Almond Butter and Blueberry Smoothie

Prep time: 5 minutes | Cook time: 10 minutes |
Serves 2

- 2 cups frozen blueberries
- 1¾ cups unsweetened almond milk
- 1 cup frozen spinach
- ¼ cup almond butter
- ½ cup ice

1. In a blender, combine the blueberries, almond milk, spinach, and almond butter. Process until smooth.
2. Add the ice, and blend again until smooth.

PER SERVING

Calories: 324 | Fat: 22g | Carbs: 29g | Fiber: 10g | Protein: 11g

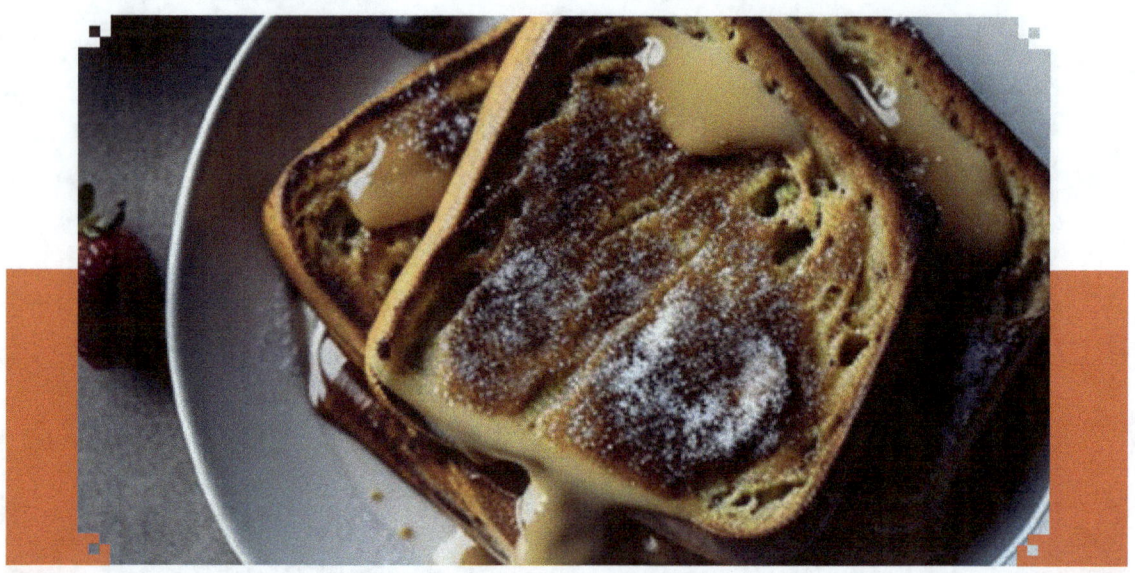

Almost-Instant Oatmeal

Prep time: 5 minutes | Cook time: 10 minutes | Serves 2

- 2 cups vanilla soy milk, plus more if needed
- ¾ cup oat bran
- 2 tablespoons natural peanut butter
- 2 teaspoons pure maple syrup
- ¼ teaspoon ground cinnamon
- 1 banana, sliced, divided
- 1 tablespoon hemp seeds, divided

1. Heat the soy milk in a large pot over high heat. Add the oat bran, peanut butter, maple syrup, and cinnamon, stirring as you go. When it starts to boil, turn the heat down to medium-low.
2. Divided the oatmeal between two bowls. Top each with half of the sliced banana and hemp seeds.

PER SERVING

Calories: 354 | Fat: 15g | Carbs: 54g | Fiber: 9g | Protein: 18g

Classic French Toast

Prep time: 10 minutes | Cook time: 3 minutes | Serves 2

- 2 large egg whites
- 2 tablespoons fat-free milk
- ¼ teaspoon vanilla extract
- ⅛ teaspoon ground cinnamon
- 1 ½ teaspoons canola or corn oil

1. In a medium shallow bowl, whisk together the egg whites, milk, vanilla, and cinnamon.
2. Using a nonstick griddle over medium heat, heat the oil, swirling to coat the griddle.
3. Transfer both slices of bread to the griddle. Cook the bread for 2 to 3 minutes on each side, or until golden brown.

PER SERVING

Calories: 124 | Fat: 4.5 g | Carbs: 13 g | Fiber: 2 g | Protein: 8 g

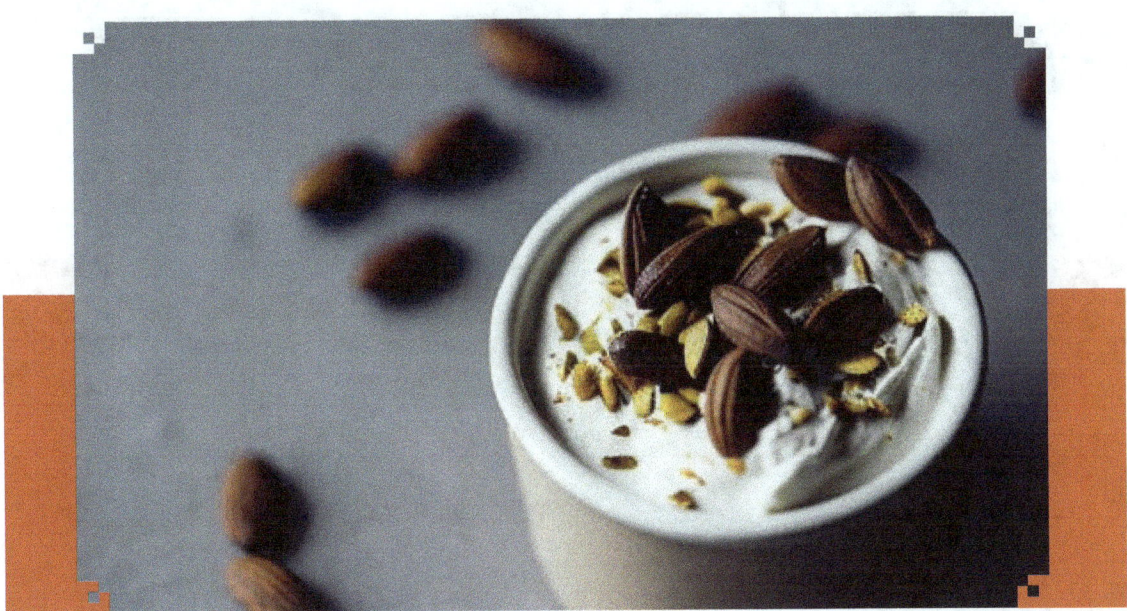

California Scrambled Eggs and Veggies

Prep time: 15 minutes | Cook time: 15 minutes | Serves 2

- 4 large eggs
- pinch salt
- ¼ cup chopped simple roasted peppers or jarred roasted red peppers (optional)
- 1 avocado, peeled, pitted, and diced

1. Crack the eggs into a large bowl. Season with salt and pepper, and whisk well.
2. In a large, nonstick skillet, melt the Better Butter over medium-low heat. Slide the arugula out of the pan and onto a plate.
3. Top with the avocado.

PER SERVING

Calories: 315 | Fat: 24g |Carbs: 11g | Fiber: 6g | Protein: 15g

Greek Yogurt Topped with Almonds

Prep time: 5 minutes | Cook time: 10 minutes | Serves 2

- ¼ teaspoon ground turmeric
- ¼ teaspoon cinnamon powder
- ⅛ teaspoon freshly ground black pepper
- ¼ cup raw almonds, sliced

1. Preheat the oven to 425°F. Line a baking sheet with parchment paper.
2. Bake for 5 to 8 minutes, until golden brown and fragrant.
3. To serve, fill each serving bowl with 1 cup of yogurt and top with the nut and seed mixture. Store nuts in an airtight container in the refrigerator for up to 5 days.

PER SERVING

Calories: 310 | Fat: 15g | Carbs: 15g | Fiber: 3g | Protein: 32g

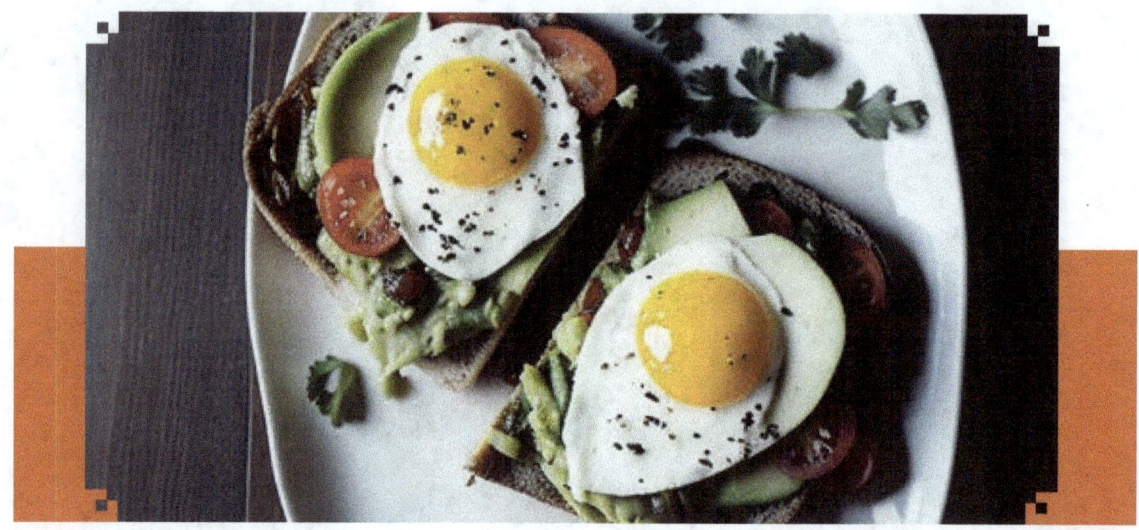

Herb and Goat Cheese Egg White Omelet

Prep time: 10 minutes | Cook time: none | Serves 2

- 2 teaspoons canola or corn oil
- 3 large egg whites
- 1 large egg
- ⅛ teaspoon salt
- Pepper to taste

1. In a large nonstick skillet, heat the oil over medium-high heat, swirling to coat the bottom.
2. Sprinkle or spread the goat cheese over half the omelet. Sprinkle with the pepper. Using a spatula, carefully fold the half with no filling over the other half. Gently slide the omelet onto a large plate. Cut the omelet in half. Transfer half to a separate large plate.

PER SERVING

Calories: 122 | Fat: 8.5 g | Carbs: 1 g | Fiber: 0 g | Protein: 10

Avocado and Tomato Toasts

Prep time: 5 minutes | Cook time: 5 minutes | Serves 2

- 1 tablespoon extra-virgin olive oil
- 2 large eggs
- 1 ripe avocado, pitted, peeled, and sliced
- 2 whole-wheat bread slices, toasted
- salt
- freshly ground black pepper
- pinch red pepper flakes
- 1 large tomato, thinly sliced

1. In a skillet, heat the oil over medium heat.
2. Carefully crack the eggs into the skillet, and fry for 3 to 4 minutes. Flip, and cook for 30 seconds, or until cooked to your desired doneness. Turn off the heat. Remove the eggs from the skillet.
3. Top with the tomato slices and eggs.

PER SERVING

Calories: 411 |Fat: 28g | Carbs: 29g | Fiber: 12g | Protein: 14g

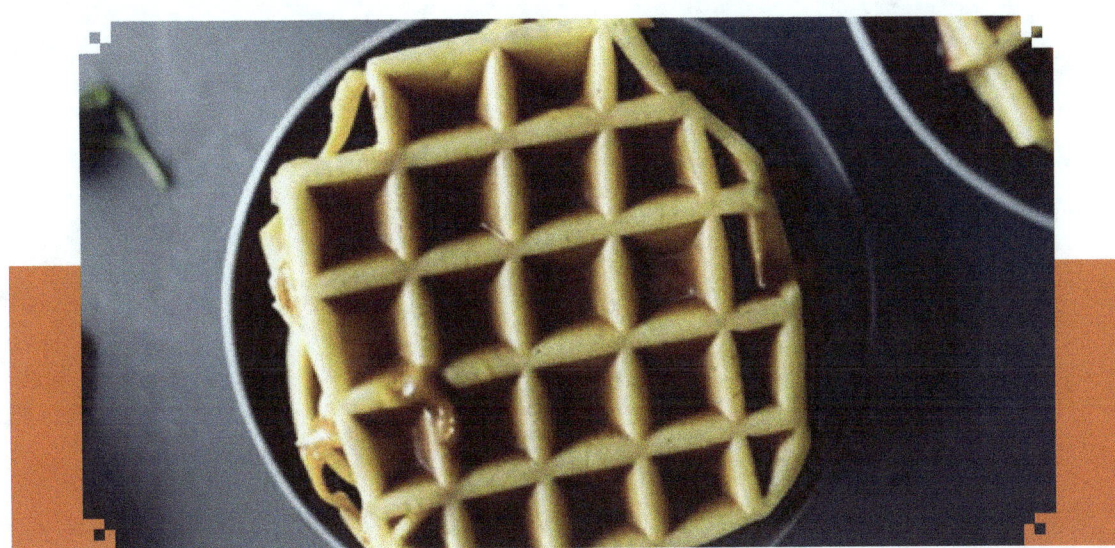

Kiwi Clementine Smoothie

Prep time: 10 minutes | Cook time: none | Serves 2

- 2 kiwis, peeled and diced
- 2 clementines, peeled and diced
- 1 banana, peeled and sliced
- 1 cup coconut water
- 2 cups baby spinach
- ¼ cup Greek yogurt

1. Ready all the fruits and vegetables, then put them in a blender.
2. Toss in the rest of the smoothie ingredients.
3. Hit the pulse button to blend the smoothie until smooth.
4. Chill the smoothie for 2 hours in the refrigerator.
5. Serve chilled and fresh.

PER SERVING

Calories: 182 | Fat: 1.6g | Carbs: 40.1g | Fiber: 7.1g | Protein: 6.4g

Omelet Waffles

Prep time: 10 minutes | Cook time: 5 minutes | Serves 2

- 4 eggs
- A pinch of black pepper
- 2 tablespoons ham, chopped
- ¼ cup low-fat cheddar, shredded
- 2 tablespoons parsley, chopped
- Cooking spray

1. Combine the eggs with pepper, ham, cheese and parsley in a bowl and whisk effectively.
2. Grease your waffle iron with cooking spray, add the egg mix, cook for 4-5 minutes.
3. Divide the waffles between plates and serve them for breakfast.
4. Enjoy!

PER SERVING

Calories: 200 | Fat: 7g | Carbs: 29g | Fiber: 3g | Protein: 3g

Chapter 5

Snack Oasis

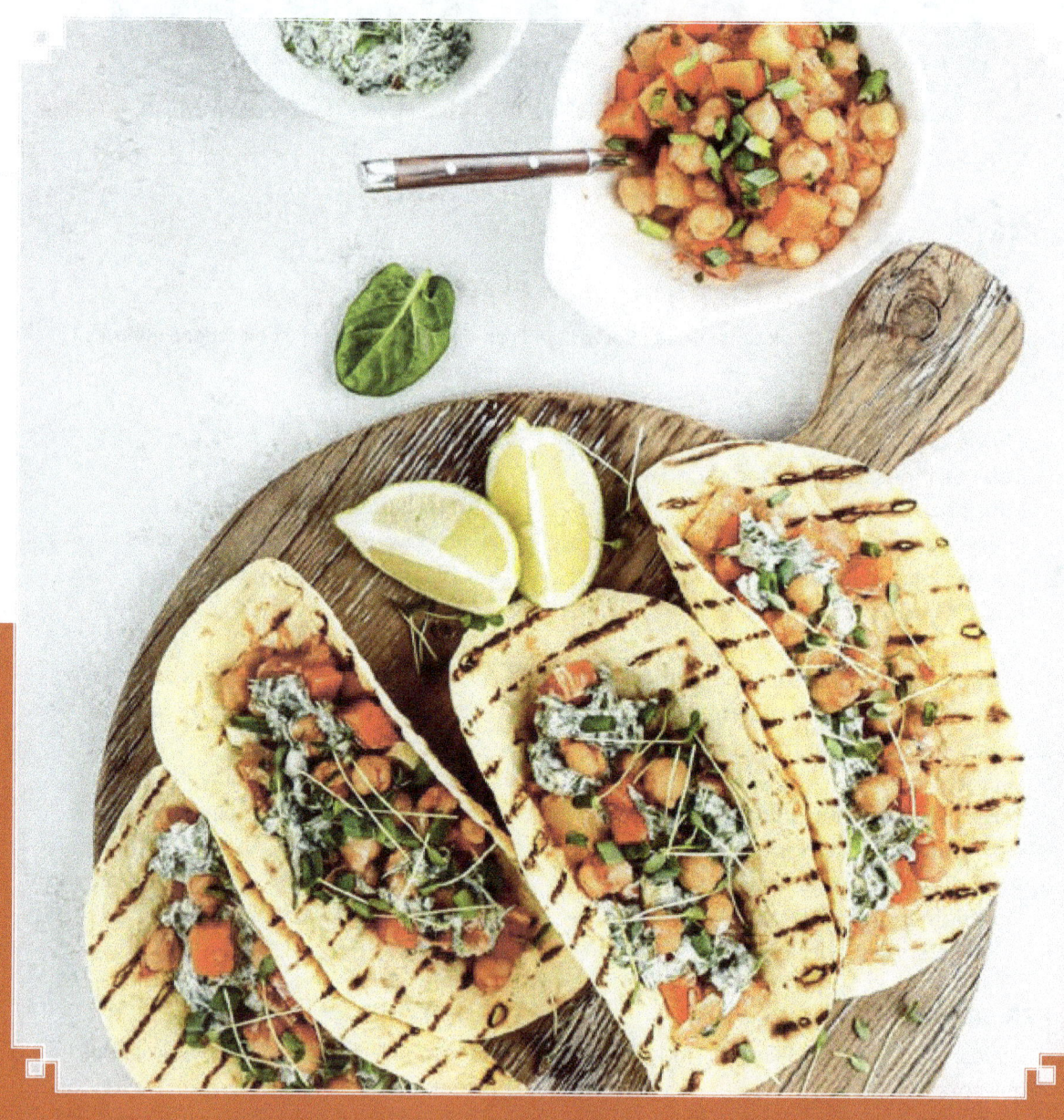

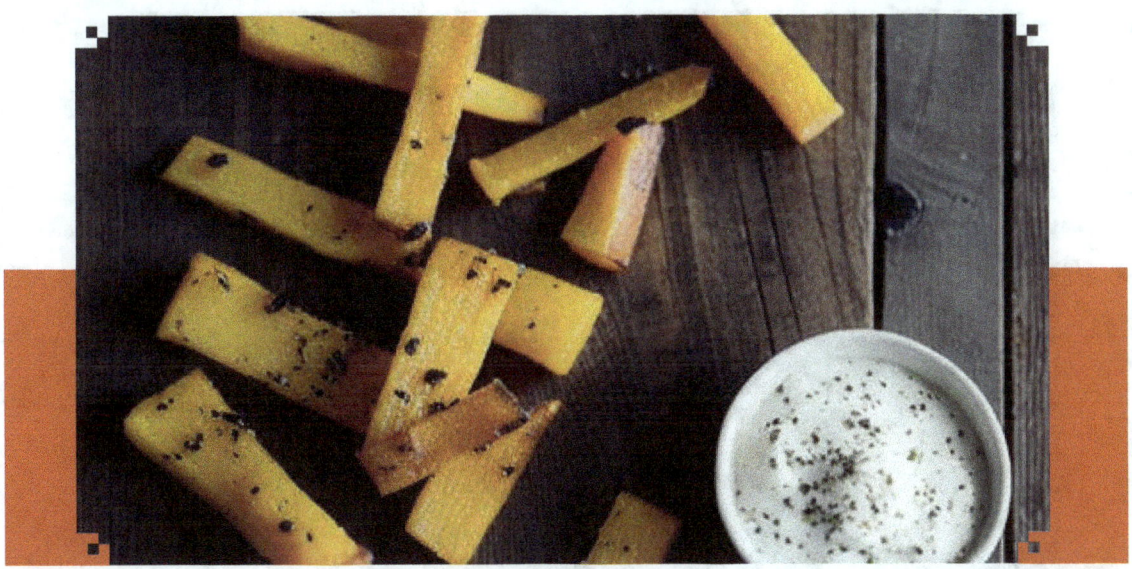

Butter Crepes with a Hint of Citrus

Prep time: 10 minutes | Cook time: 4 minutes | Serves 2

- 1 ½ cups sifted all-purpose flour
- ¾ cup fat-free milk
- ¾ cup cold water
- 2 large egg whites
- 1 tablespoon sugar
- 2 to 3 tablespoons water, as needed

1. Cooking spray (butter flavor preferred)
2. In a large mixing bowl, using an electric mixer on high, beat together the batter ingredients except the water for about 1 minute, or until smooth. The batter will be thin. Cover tightly with plastic wrap and refrigerate for 2 hours to one day.
3. Line a plate with paper towels.

PER SERVING

Calories: 94 | Fat: 2.0 g | Carbs: 15 g | Fiber: 1 g | Protein: 3 g

Butternut Squash Fries

Prep time: 10 minutes | Cook time: 10 minutes | Serves 2

- ½ medium butternut squash
- ½ tablespoon olive oil
- ½ tablespoon fresh thyme, chopped
- ½ tablespoon fresh rosemary, chopped
- ¼ teaspoon salt

1. Preheat the oven to 400°F.
2. Peel the squash and slice it into 3-inch-long and ½-inch wide pieces.
3. Place the pieces in a large bowl and toss with the oil, thyme, salt, and rosemary.
4. Spread the squash on the baking sheet and bake for 8 minutes.
5. Toss the fries well and bake again for 2 minutes or more until golden brown.
6. Serve.

PER SERVING

Calories: 117 | Fat: 19g | Carbs: 29g | Fiber: 1.8g | Protein: 2.5g

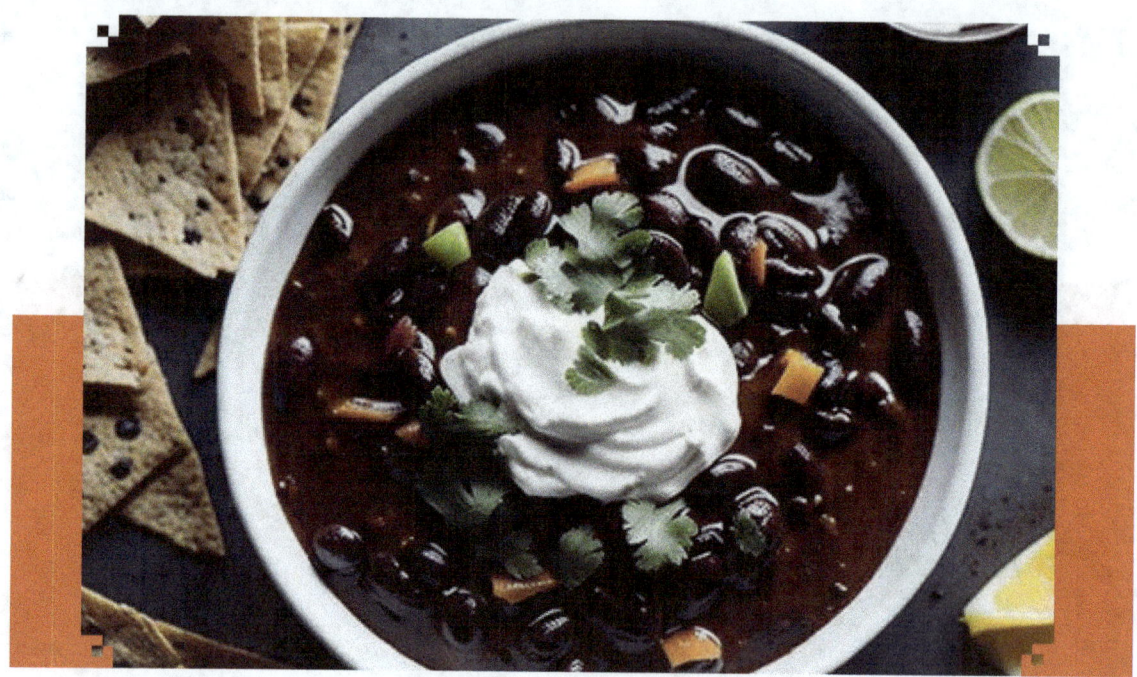

Caprese Skewers

Prep time: 5 minutes |Cook time: 5 minute
|Serves 2

- 12 red tomatoes
- 2 red bell peppers
- 12 basil leaves
- 8 (1-inch) pieces of ricotta cheese
- ¼ cup italian vinaigrette

1. Thread the following onto each of four wooden skewers: 1 tomato, 1 basil leaf, 1 mozzarella cube, 1 tomato, and 1 red bell pepper 1 basil leaf, 1 cheese cube, 1 basil leaf, and 1 tomato
2. If desired, serve with vinaigrette for dipping.

PER SERVING:

Calories: 338| Fat: 24g| Carbs: 6g| Fiber: 0g |Protein: 25g

Black Bean Dip

Prep time: 10 minutes | Cook time: 2 minutes |
Serves 2

- 1 (15 ounces) can black beans, drained, with liquid reserved
- ¼ cup plain Greek yogurt
- Black pepper, to taste

1. Combine beans, peppers, and yogurt in a food processor or blender and process until smooth.
2. Add some of the bean liquid, 1 tablespoon at a time, for a thinner consistency.
3. Season to taste with black pepper.
4. Serve.

PER SERVING

Calories: 70 | Fat: 1 g | Carbs: 11 g | Fiber:4 g | Protein: 5 g

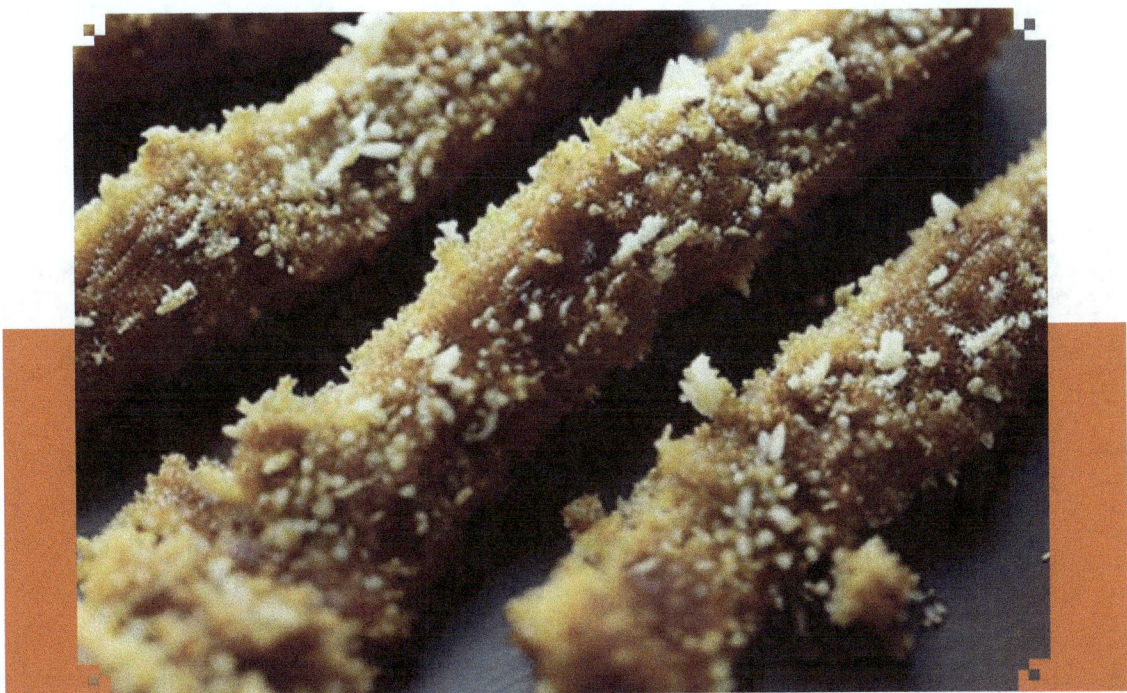

Garlicky Green Beans

Prep time: 5 minutes | Cook time: 10 minutes | Serves 2

- 2 garlic cloves, minced
- ½ tablespoon olive oil
- ½ pound fresh green beans, trimmed and cut-into 1-inch pieces
- Fresh ground black pepper to taste

1. Take a large frying pan, heat oil over medium heat and fry garlic for about a minute.
2. Add green beans, salt and black pepper and cook for about 8 minutes.
3. Serve hot and enjoy!

PER SERVING

Calories: 90 | Fat: 4.9g | Carbs: 11.5g | Fiber: 5.2g | Protein: 2.9g

Zucchini Sticks

Prep time: 10 minutes | Cook time: 20 minutes | Serves 2

- 3 medium zucchinis, sliced into sticks
- 1 cup whole-wheat breadcrumbs
- ½ cup Parmesan cheese, grated
- 1 egg
- ¼ teaspoon salt
- ¼ teaspoon black pepper

1. Preheat oven to 400° F.
2. Line a baking pan with parchment paper set aside.
3. Arrange on the baking sheet, then bake until crispy and golden brown.

PER SERVING

Calories: 128 | Fat: 7g | Carbs: 10g | Fiber: 1g | Protein: 6g

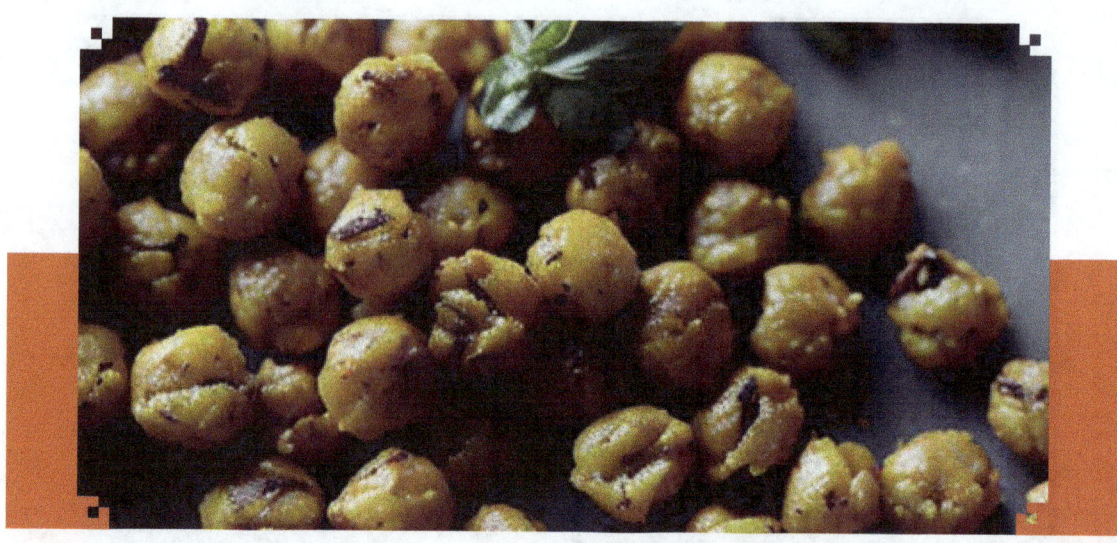

Stuffed Sweet Potatoes with Pistachios

Prep time: 5 minutes | Cook time: 20 minutes | Serves 2

- 2 small sweet potatoes (each about 5 inches long), skin well scrubbed
- ½ cup unsalted pistachios
- 2 teaspoons grated parmesan cheese
- juice of ½ lemon
- 2 sprigs fresh thyme

1. Prick the sweet potatoes all over with a fork. Being careful of the steam that will release, open the potatoes wide, and mash the flesh with a fork.
2. Add the pistachio mixture to the asparagus and combine well. Season with salt and pepper, if desired.
3. Scoop half of the mixture into each sweet potato and garnish with fresh thyme.

PER SERVING

Calories: 409 | Fat: 19 g | Carbs: 52 g | Fiber: 10 g | Protein: 13 g

Roasted Chickpeas

Prep time: 5 minutes | Cook time: 30 minutes | Serves 2

- 1 (15-ounce can) chickpeas, drained and rinsed
- ½ teaspoon olive oil
- 2 teaspoons of your favorite herbs or spice blend
- ¼ teaspoon salt

1. Preheat the oven to 400°F.
2. In a medium bowl, gently toss the chickpeas and olive oil until combined. Sprinkle the mixture with the herbs and salt and toss again.
3. Place the chickpeas back on the baking sheet and spread in an even layer.
4. Bake for 30 to 40 minutes, until crunchy and golden brown. Stir halfway through.
5. Serve.

PER SERVING

Calories: 175 | Fat: 3g | Carbs: 29g | Fiber: 11g | Protein: 11g

Chapter 6

Soup & Salad Symphony

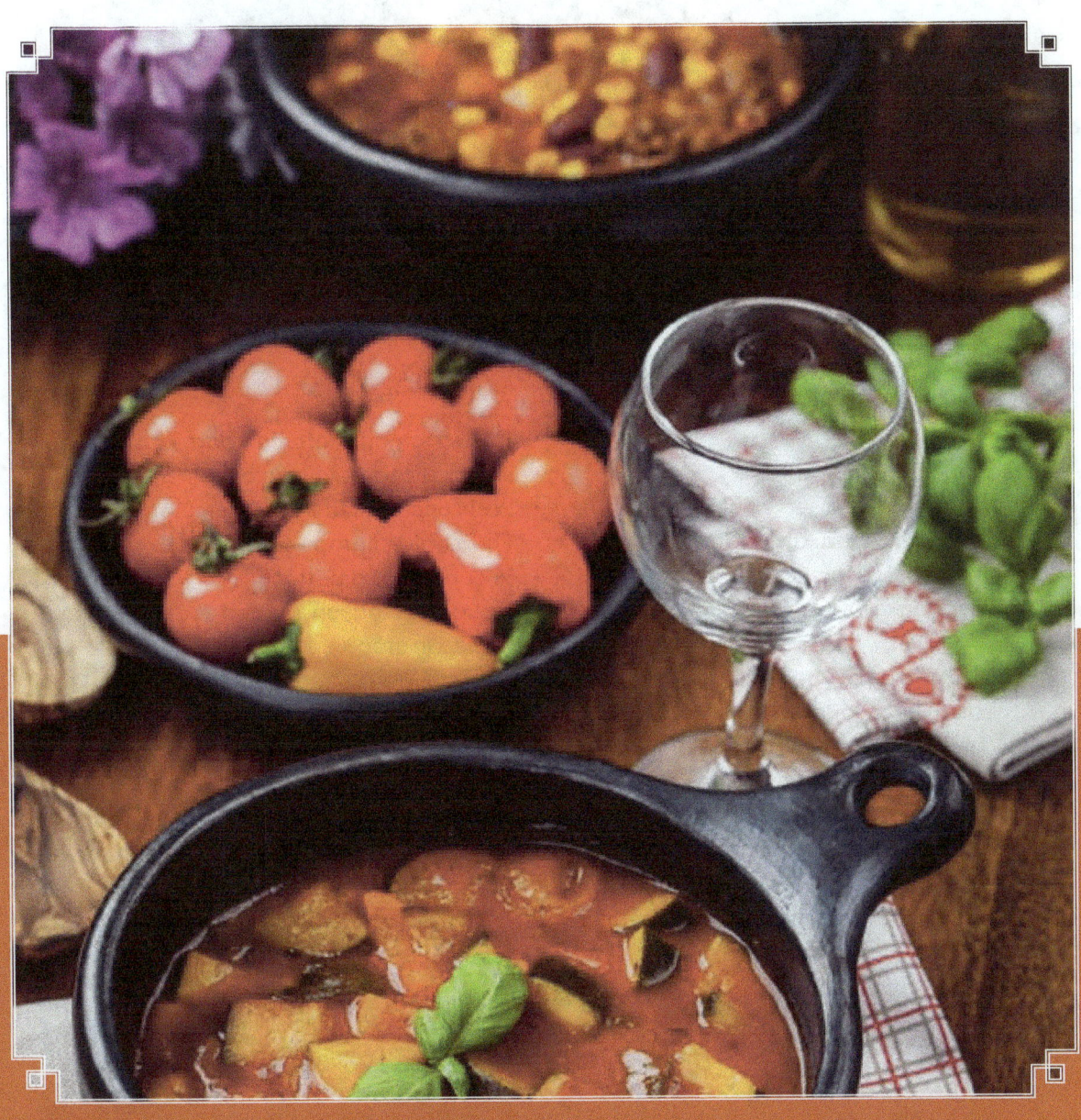

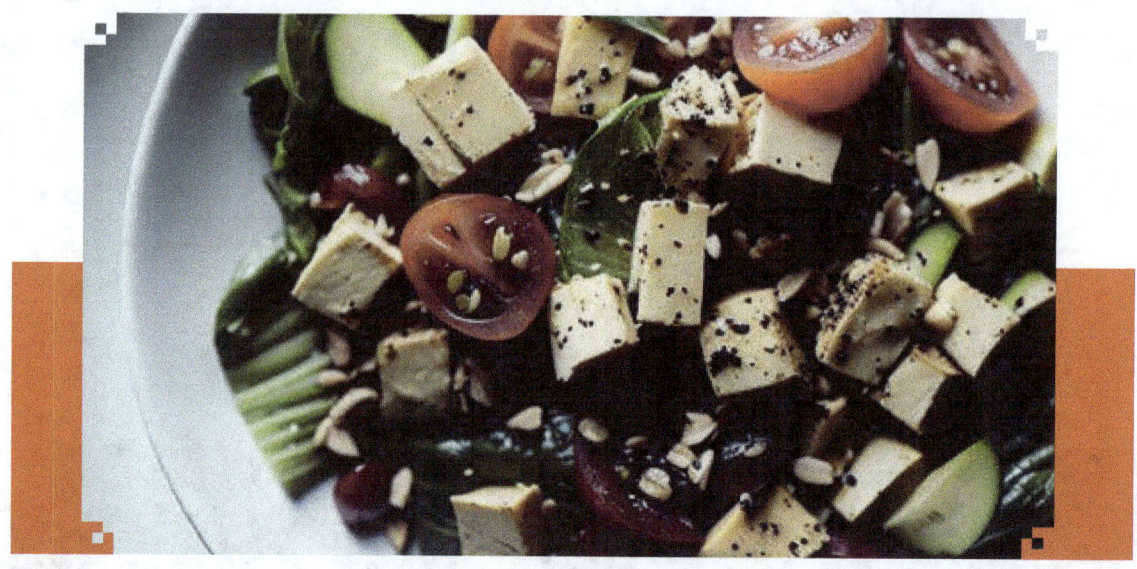

Warm Balsamic Beet Salad with Sunflower Seeds

Prep time: 10 minutes | Cook time: 15 minutes | Serves 2

- 2 teaspoons avocado oil
- 3 medium whole beets, including greens and roots, chopped, divided
- 1 tablespoon balsamic vinegar
- 1 tablespoon sunflower seeds

1. In a medium pot, heat the oil over medium heat for about 2 minutes.
2. Add the beet roots and cook, covered, for 5 to 7 minutes, until they are fork-tender but not soft.
3. In a large mixing bowl, combine balsamic vinegar, sunflower seeds, and the beet container in the refrigerator for up to 3 days.

PER SERVING

Calories: 111 | Fat: 5g |Carbs: 14g | Fiber: 6g | Protein: 4g

Easy Basic Table Salad

Prep time: 5 minutes |Cook time: 2 minutes |Serves 2

- 1 head romaine lettuce coarsely chopped
- ½ cup sliced yellow onion
- ½–1 zucchini, cut in quarters
- 1 cup halved grape tomatoes
- ⅔ cup almond butter
- 1 cup pressed and diced extra-firm tofu added in step 1
- 1 peach, pitted and diced
- sprinkle of nutritional yeast
- toasted sesame

1. Mix the lettuce, onion, zucchini, tofu, peach, nutritional yeast, sesame and tomatoes in a large bowl.
2. Top with the dressing, then toss to coat.

PER SERVING:

Calories: 648| Fat: 49.5g| Carbs: 42.4g| Protein: 21.8g | Fiber: 0g

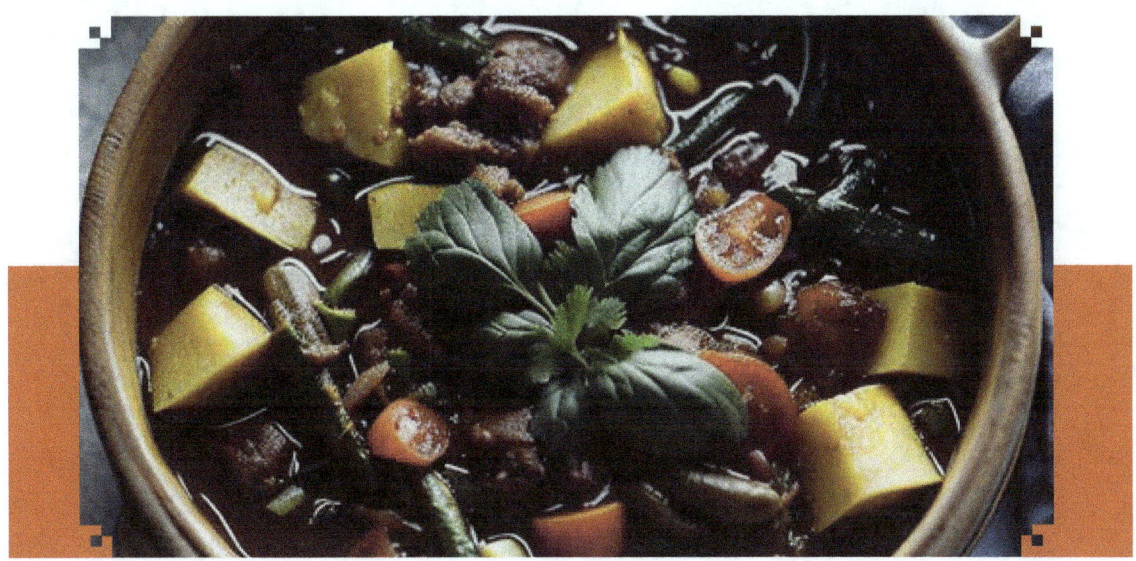

Salmon & Veggie Soup

Prep time: 10 minutes | Cook time: 30 minutes | Serves 2

- ½ shallot, chopped
- ½ Jalapeno pepper, chopped
- 1 tablespoon olive oil
- 1 garlic clove, minced
- 2½ cups low-sodium vegetable broth
- Fresh ground black pepper to taste

1. Take a large soup pan, heat oil over medium heat and fry shallot and garlic for about two to three minutes.
2. Add cabbage and bell peppers and fry them for about three to four minutes.
3. Stir in the cilantro, lemon juice and black pepper and cook for about one to two minutes.
4. Serve hot and enjoy!

PER SERVING

Calories: 250 | Fat: 13.2g | Carbs: 11.7g | Fiber: 3.1g | Protein: 23.8g

Bean, Squash, and Tomato Stew

Prep time: 10 minutes | Cook time: 40 minutes | Serves 2

- 2 tablespoons extra-virgin olive oil
- 1 small red onion, thinly sliced
- 5 cups zucchini, about 2 large zucchini, chopped
- 2 celery stalks, sliced
- 4 cloves garlic, sliced
- ¼ cup chopped fresh cilantro

1. In a large saucepan, heat the olive oil over medium-low heat. Add the onion, and translucent, 8 to 10 minutes. Add the garlic and cook for 1 minute.
2. Add the beans and 2 cups water, cover, and simmer for another 15 to 20 the flavors.
3. Serve garnished with fresh cilantro.

PER SERVING

Calories: 442 | Fat: 14 g | Carbs: 65 g | Fiber: 19 g |Protein: 17 g

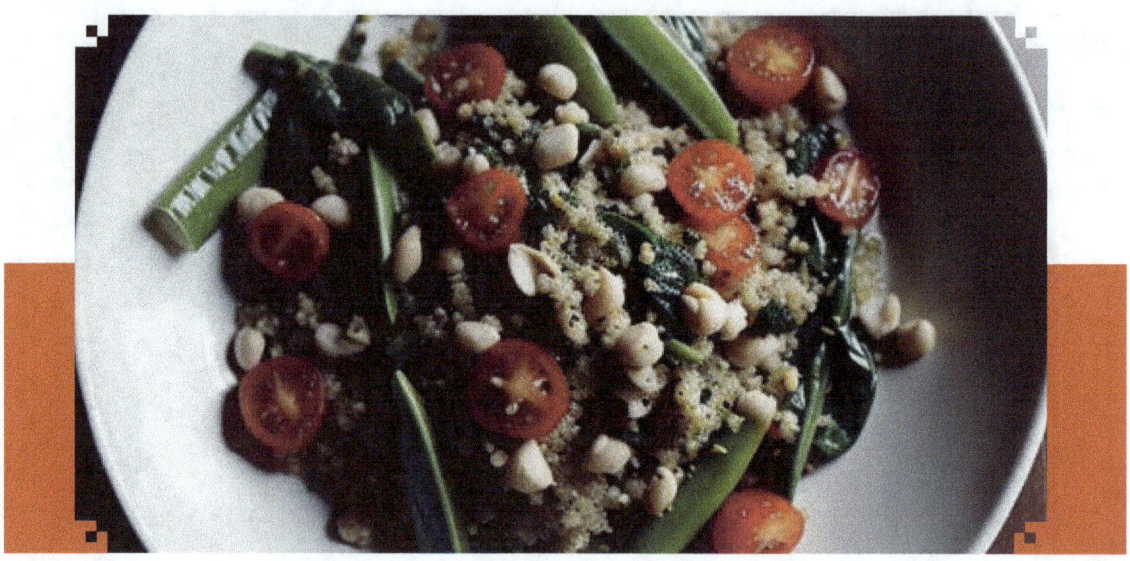

Hearty Vegetable Stew

Prep time: 15 minutes |Cook time: 25 minutes |Serves 2

- 2 teaspoons olive oil
- 2 celery stalks, chopped
- ½ sweet onion, peeled and chopped
- 1 teaspoon minced garlic
- 3 cups low-sodium vegetable broth
- 1 cup chopped tomatoes
- 1 tablespoon chopped fresh parsley, for garnish

1. In a large saucepan, warm the olive oil over medium-high heat.
2. Add celery, onions, and garlic, and sauté until softened, about 4 minutes.
3. Season with salt and pepper.
4. Serve topped with Parmesan cheese and parsley.

PER SERVING:

Calories: 270| Fat: 8g| Carbs: 35g| Protein: 17g | Fiber: 2g

Quinoa and Spinach Power Salad

Prep time: 5 minutes | Cook time: 10 minutes | Serves 2

- ½ cup quinoa, rinsed and drained
- 2 cups spinach, finely chopped
- 1 medium tomato, diced
- 1 cup sugar snap peas
- ½ cup diced cucumbers
- ¼ teaspoon freshly ground black pepper

1. In a medium saucepan, combine the until the quinoa has absorbed all of the water, 10 to 15 minutes.
2. In a small bowl, whisk together the lemon juice, olive oil, salt, and pepper. Pour over the quinoa and vegetables and toss to coat.
3. Portion into 2 serving bowls.

PER SERVING

Calories: 439 | Fat: 20 g | Carbs: 54 g | Fiber: 10 g | Protein: 15 g

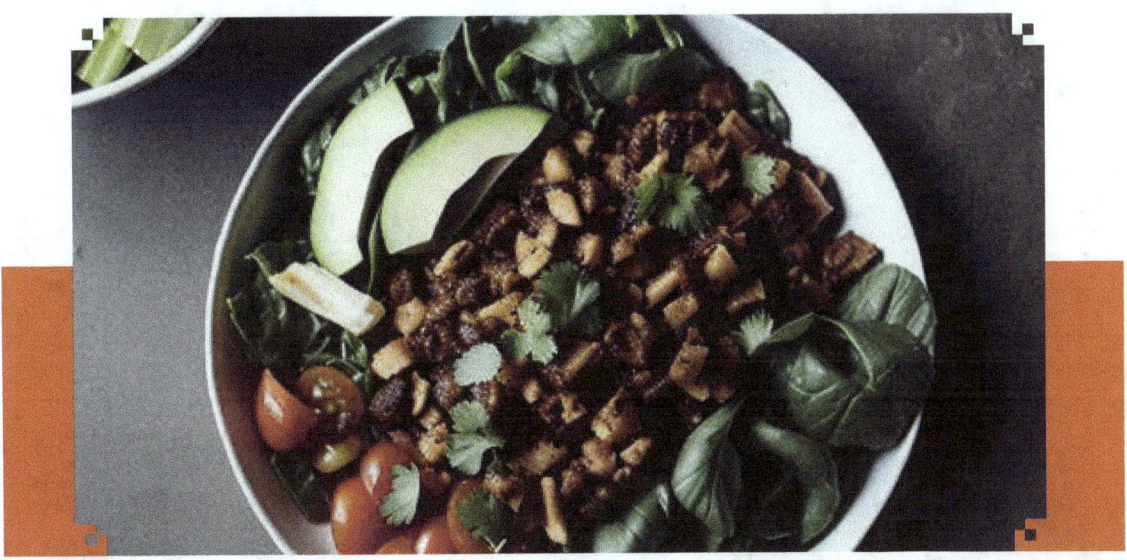

Arugula, Pumpkin Seed, and Carrot Salad

Prep time: 10 minutes | Cook time: 15 minutes | Serves 2

- ½ teaspoon thyme
- 1 teaspoon honey
- 1 teaspoon avocado oil
- 2 large carrots, cut into thin coins
- 3 tablespoons unsalted pumpkin seeds
- 4 cups arugula
- 2 teaspoons extra-virgin olive oil
- freshly ground black pepper

1. Preheat the oven to 400°F. Line a baking sheet with parchment paper.
2. Divide the arugula and carrot-and-seed mixture into two bowls for serving. Drizzle with the olive oil and add pepper to taste.

PER SERVING

Calories: 176 | Fat: 12g | Carbs: 14g | Fiber: 4g | Protein: 6g

Tempeh Taco Salad with Chile-Lime Glaze

Prep time: 5 minutes | Cook time: 5 minutes | Serves 2

- 1 teaspoon avocado oil
- ¼ red onion, diced (about ¼ cup diced)
- 1 head romaine lettuce, chopped
- 1 cup tomatoes, diced
- 1 medium cucumber, quartered
- ¼ avocado, sliced
- 2 tablespoons Chile-Lime Glaze

1. In a medium pan, heat the oil over medium-low heat and add the onion and garlic. Sauté for about 1 minute, until the onion becomes translucent.
2. Divide the romaine lettuce, tomatoes, cucumber, tempeh mixture, and avocado into two serving bowls. kept in the refrigerator.

PER SERVING

Calories: 225 |Fat: 11g | Carbs: 28g | Fiber: 7g | Protein: 7g

Chapter 7

Ocean's Bounty

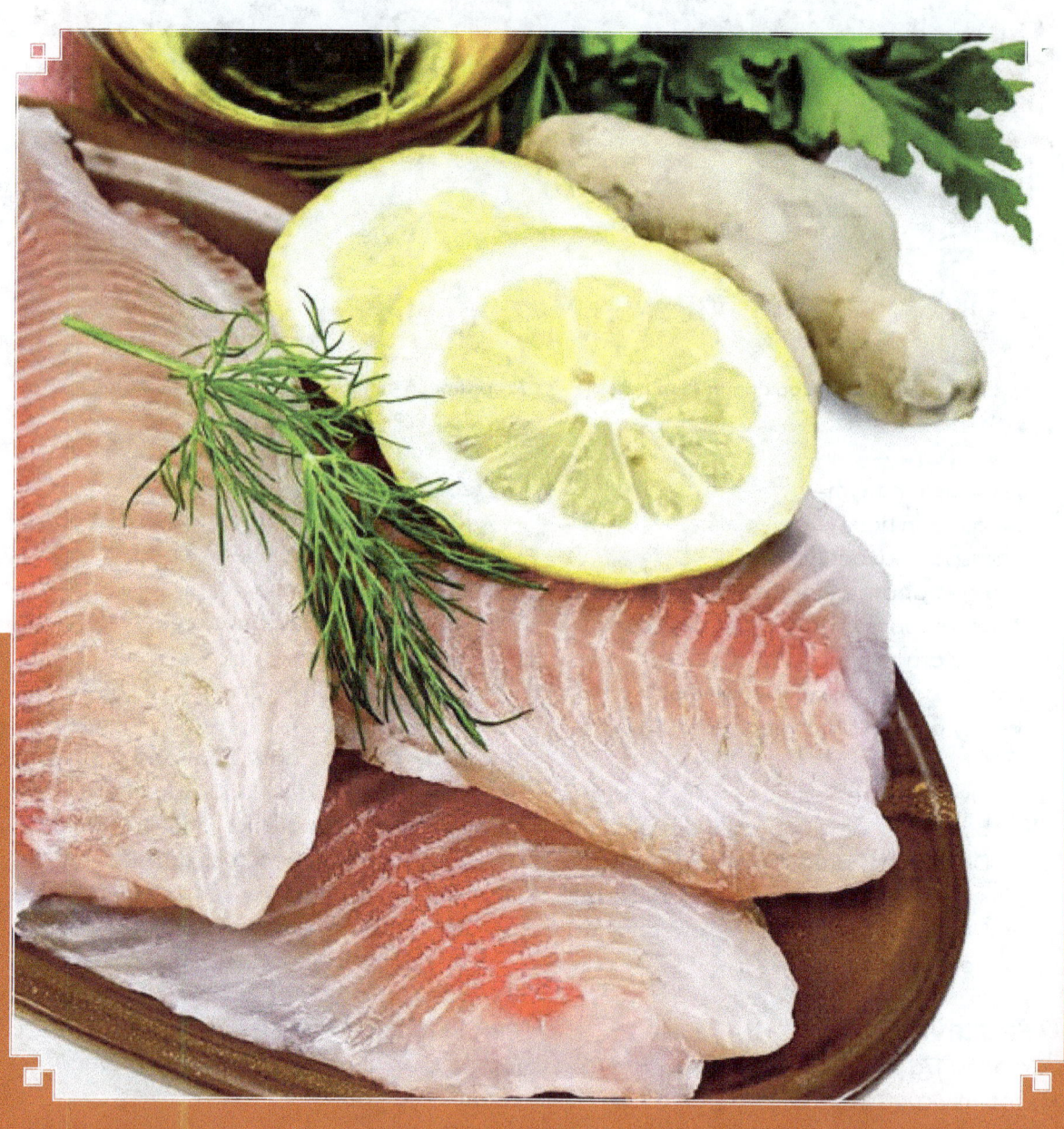

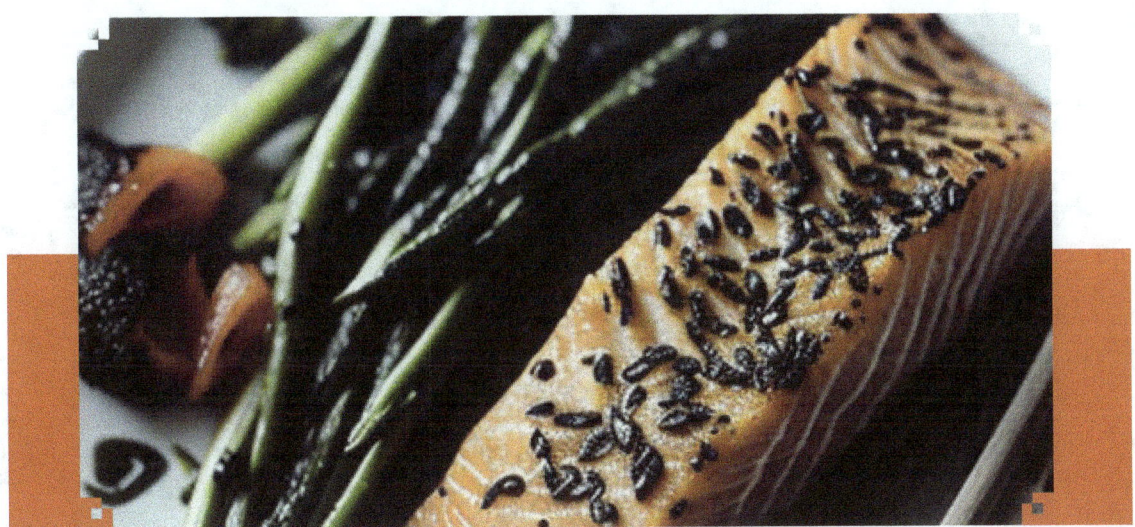

Mahi Mahi with Leeks, Ginger, and Baby Bok Choy

Prep time: 10 minutes | Cook time: 15 minutes | Serves 2

- 2 teaspoons toasted sesame oil
- 1 packed tablespoon grated ginger
- 3 bunches baby bok choy, separated
- 2 (4-ounce) mahi mahi fillets, skinned
- ¼ teaspoon freshly ground black pepper
- ¼ teaspoon garlic powder

1. Heat a 5-quart pot over medium heat, pour in the sesame oil, and add the leek. Sauté until fragrant and translucent, 1 to 2 minutes.
2. Flip the mahi mahi and add the leek, ginger, and bok choy mixture on top. Cook for another 2 to 3 minutes until the mahi mahi is cooked, flaky, and tender. Serve.

PER SERVING

Calories: 193 | Fat: 6g | Carbs: 8g | Sugars: 3g | Fiber: 5g | Protein: 24g

Sesame Salmon Fillets

Prep time: 5 minutes | Cook time: 6 minutes | Serves 2

- 1 tablespoon sesame oil
- 2 (4-ounce) salmon fillets, skin on
- 1/8 teaspoon ground ginger
- 1/8 teaspoon sea salt
- 1/8 teaspoon cracked black pepper
- 2 teaspoons black sesame seeds

1. Heat the oil in a medium pan over medium heat. Once the pan is hot, add the salmon, skin side down.
2. Top each fillet with the ginger powder, salt, pepper, and sesame seeds. Pat the seeds down softly so they stick to the fillet.
3. After about 3 to 4 minutes, turn the fillets over, and sear the other side. After 1 to 2 minutes, remove the fillets from the pan and serve immediately.

PER SERVING

Calories:319 | Fat:21 g | Carbs:2 g | Fiber:1 g | Protein:31 g

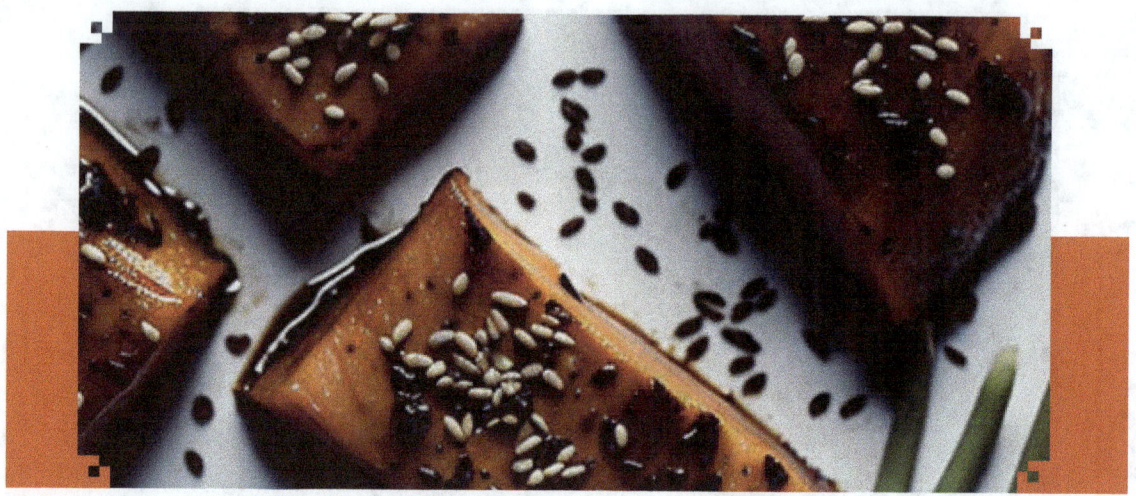

Crispy Trout with Herb

Prep time: 10 minutes |Cook time: 20 minutes |Serves 2

- 1 lb. fresh trout (2 pieces)
- 2 cups fish stock
- ¼ tsp. dried thyme, ground
- 1 tbsp. fresh parsley, chopped
- 1 tbsp. fresh mint, chopped
- 3 tbsps. olive oil
- 2 tbsps. fresh lemon juice
- 3 garlic cloves, chopped
- 1 tsp. sea salt

1. Mix mint, parsley, thyme, garlic, lemon juice, olive oil, and salt in a bowl. Stir to combine. Spread the fish and brush with the marinade. Set aside.
2. Insert the trivet into the instant pot. Seal the lid and cook on Steam mode for 15 minutes with High Pressure. Quick release and serve immediately.

PER SERVING:

Calories: 729| Fat: 45.46g| Carbs: 3.66g| Protein: 72.49g

Ginger Sesame Salmon

Prep time: 15 minutes |Cook time: 5 minutes |Serves 2

- 4 ounces salmon
- 1/8 cup low-sodium soy sauce
- 2 tablespoons of balsamic vinegar
- ½ teaspoon sesame oil
- 2-inch chunk ginger, peeled and grated
- 1 garlic clove, minced
- 1 teaspoon flavorless oil
- 1 teaspoon sesame seeds
- 1 teaspoon green onion, minced

1. Combine the soy sauce, balsamic vinegar, sesame oil, garlic, and ginger in a glass dish. Place the salmon in the container. Cover and marinate for 15 - 60 minutes in the fridge.
2. In a nonstick skillet, heat 1 teaspoon of oil. Serve immediately. Garnish with green onion.

PER SERVING:

Calories: 218| Fat: 13.5g| Carbs: 6.5g| Protein: 17g | Fiber: 2.5g

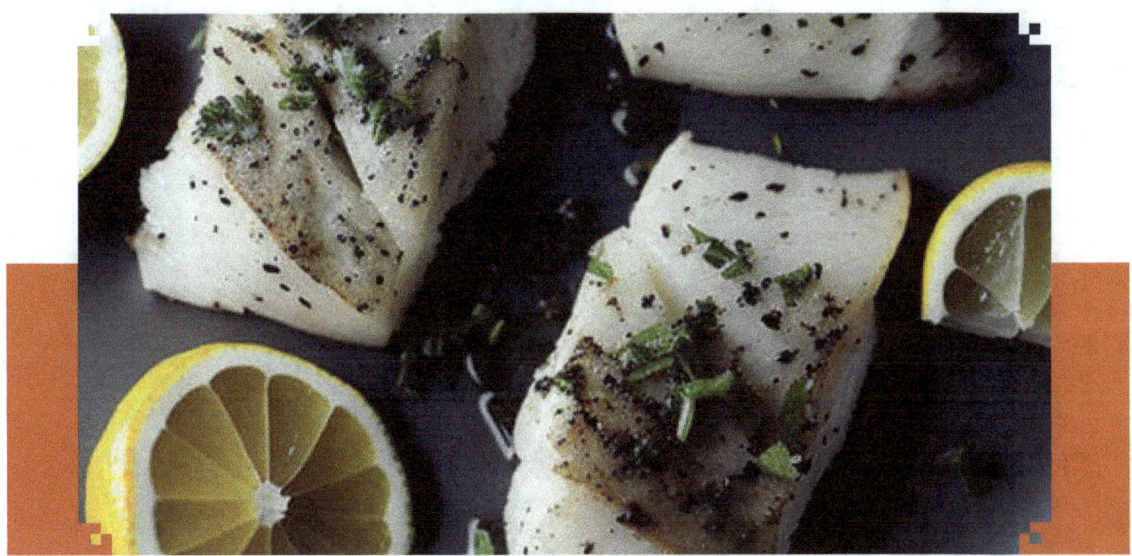

Fresh Salmon Salad Pita Pocket

Prep time: 10 minutes | Cook time: none | Serves 2

- 8 ounces cooked fresh salmon
- 1 green onion, finely chopped
- 1 celery stalk, finely chopped
- 2 tablespoons plain fat-free yogurt
- 2 teaspoons lemon juice
- 1 teaspoon chopped fresh dill
- Freshly ground pepper

1. In a medium bowl, flake cooked salmon with a fork.
2. Mix in green onion, celery, bell pepper, yogurt, lemon juice, dill, and pepper. Combine well.
3. Fill four pita halves evenly with salmon salad and shredded spinach, and serve.

PER SERVING

Calories: 308 | Fat: 8.9 g | Carbs: 30.4 g | Fiber: 5 g | Protein: 28.8 g

Herbed White Sea Bass

Prep time: 10 minutes | Cook time: 10 minutes | Serves 2

- 2 white sea bass fillets, each 4 ounces
- 1 tablespoon lemon juice
- 1 teaspoon garlic, minced
- ¼ teaspoon herb seasoning blend
- Ground black pepper, to taste

1. Preheat the broiler and place its rack about 4 inches below the heat source.
2. Grease a baking pan with cooking spray.
3. Place the fish fillets in the baking pan.
4. Add the lemon juice, pepper, herbed seasoning, and garlic on top of the fish.
5. Place the baking pan in the broiler.
6. Cook for 10 minutes.
7. Serve warm.

PER SERVING

Calories: 125 | Fat: 14g | Carbs: 1g | Fiber: 0.3g | Protein: 21g

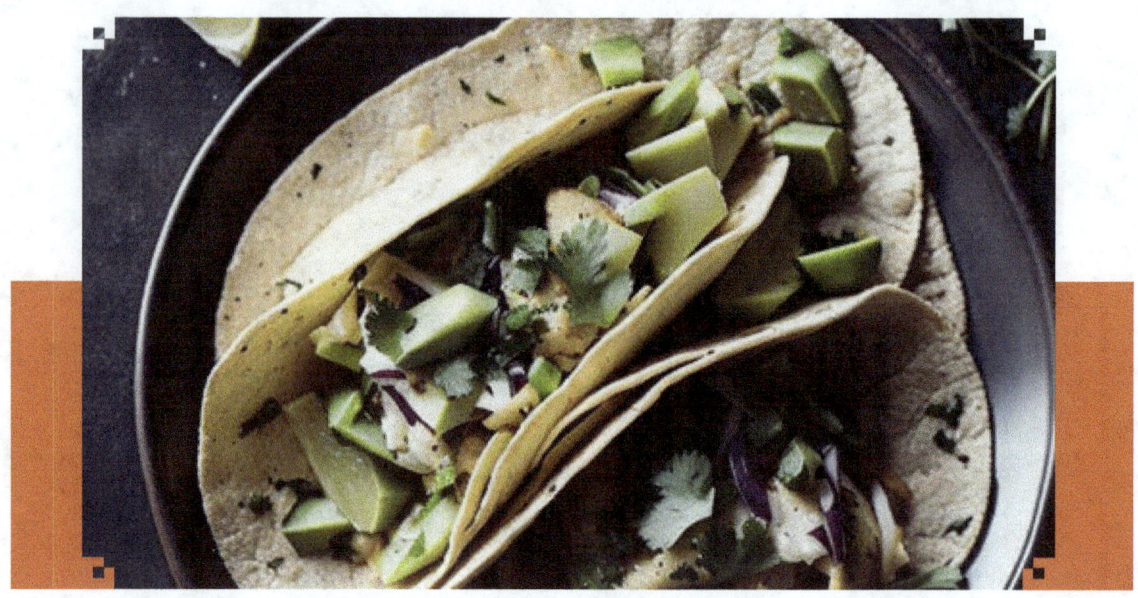

Avocado and Tuna Salad Sandwich

Prep time: 10 minutes | Cook time: 10 minutes | Serves 2

- 1 (5-ounce) can water-packed tuna, drained
- 2 scallions, green and white parts, minced
- juice of ½ lemon
- 2 tablespoons extra-virgin olive oil
- ¼ teaspoon salt
- ¼ teaspoon freshly ground black pepper
- 4 whole-wheat bread slices

1. In a small bowl, combine the tuna, avocado, scallions, lemon juice, oil, salt, and pepper.
2. Divide the tuna mixture onto 2 bread slices. Top with the remaining 2 bread slices.

PER SERVING

Calories: 518 | Fat: 32g | Carbs: 41g | Fiber: 13g | Protein: 23g

Haddock Tacos with Cabbage Slaw

Prep time: 10 minutes | Cook time: 5 minutes | Serves 2

- 1 teaspoon ground cumin
- ½ teaspoon chili powder
- ⅛ teaspoon salt
- 2 tablespoons fresh lime juice
- 3 teaspoons extra-virgin olive oil
- 2 (6-inch) whole-wheat tortillas, warmed

1. In a small bowl, combine the cumin, chili powder, salt, and pepper. Add the haddock and toss to coat.
2. Divide the fish between the warmed tortillas and top with the cabbage avocado mixture. Serve garnished with fresh cilantro.

PER SERVING

Calories: 368 | Fat: 16 g | Carbs: 22 g | Fiber: 7 g | Protein: 32 g

Chapter 8

Poultry Palate

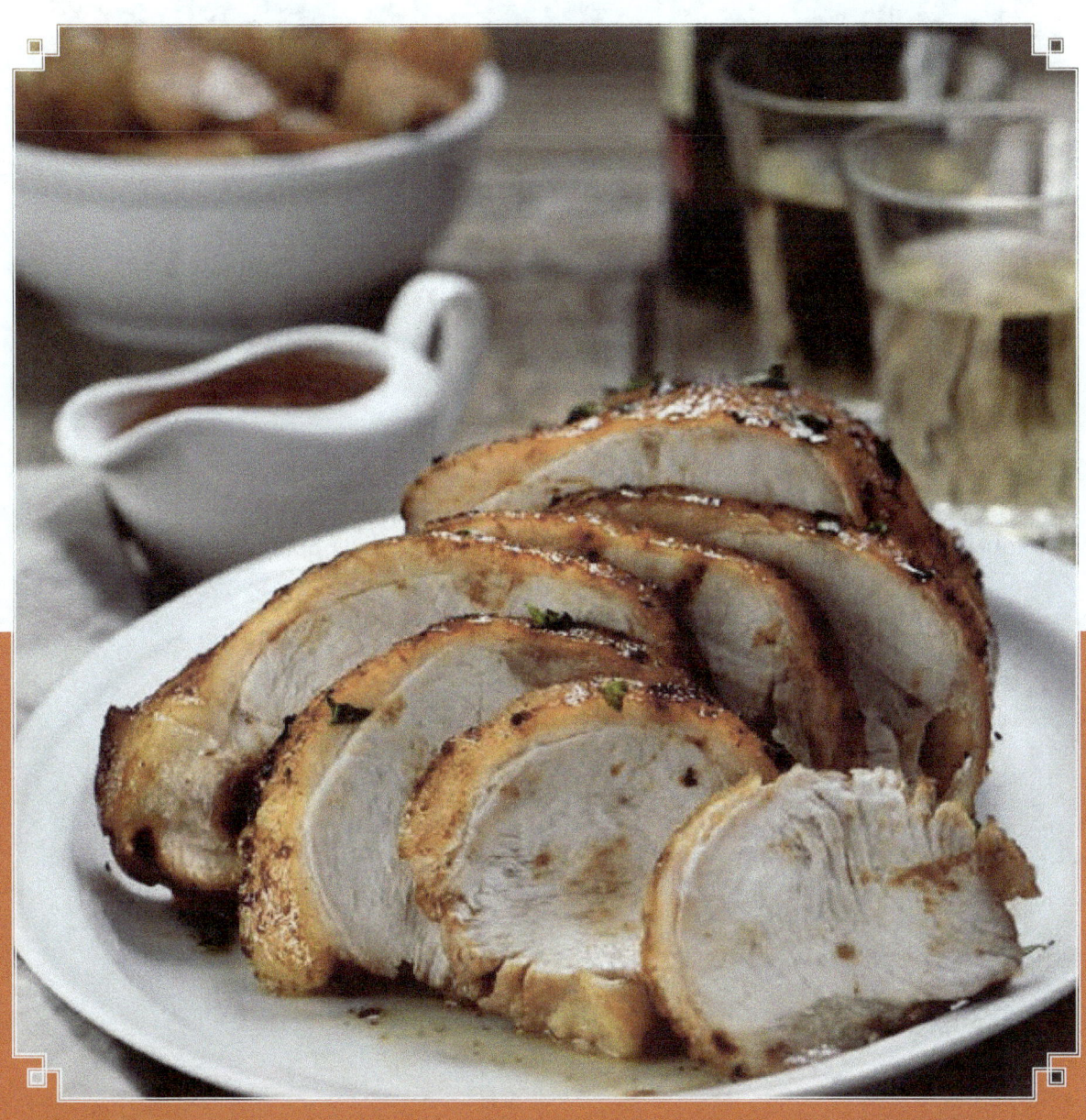

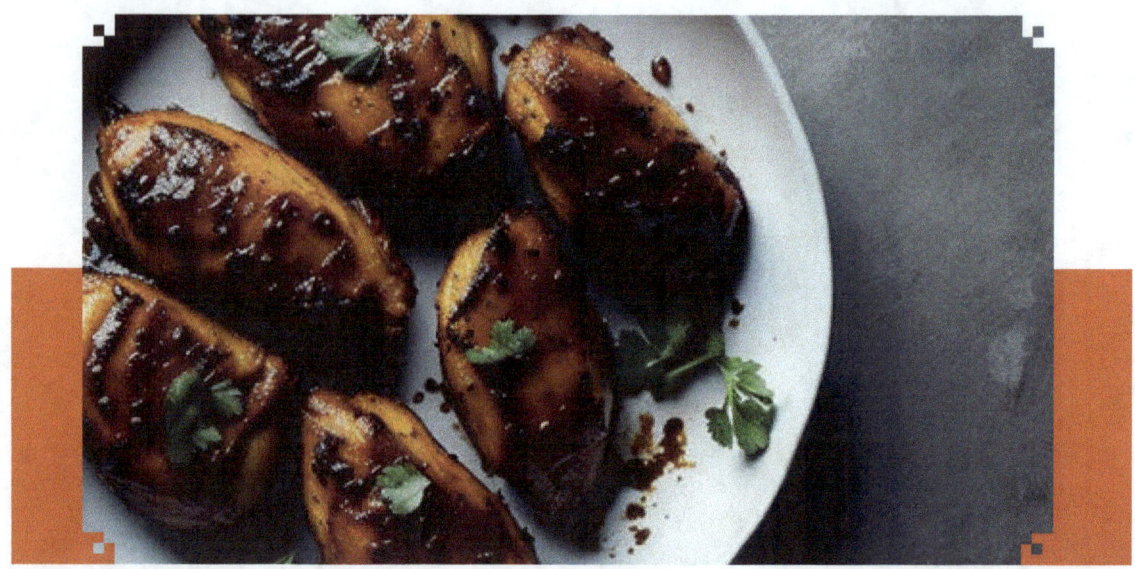

Blueberry, Pistachio, and Parsley Chicken

Prep time: 5 minutes | Cook time: 25 minutes | Serves 2

- ½ cup blueberries
- ¼ cup chopped fresh parsley
- 2 tablespoons balsamic vinegar
- ¼ teaspoon freshly ground black pepper
- 2 (4-ounce) pieces of chicken

1. Preheat the oven to 375°F. Line a baking dish with parchment paper.
2. In a medium mixing bowl, mix the blueberries, pistachios, parsley, vinegar, and pepper until well combined.
3. Put the chicken in the baking dish and pour the blueberry mixture on top. Store in the refrigerator in an airtight container for up to 3 days.

PER SERVING

Calories: 212 | Fat: 7g | Carbs: 11g | Fiber: 2g | Protein: 27g

Spicy Chicken

Prep time: 10 minutes |Cook time: 18 minutes |Serves 2

- 2 chicken breasts, boneless
- 1 1/2 tsp chili powder
- 3 tbsp sriracha sauce
- 1/4 tsp smoked paprika
- 1 tbsp brown sugar
- 1 tsp onion powder
- 1 tsp garlic powder
- salt

1. Preheat your air fryer to 350 F.
2. Add chicken and remaining ingredients into the large mixing bowl and mix until well coated.
3. Cover bowl and place in refrigerator for 6 hours.
4. Serve and enjoy.

PER SERVING:

Calories: 433| Fat: 25.3g| Carbs: 8g| Protein: 43g | Fiber: 6 g

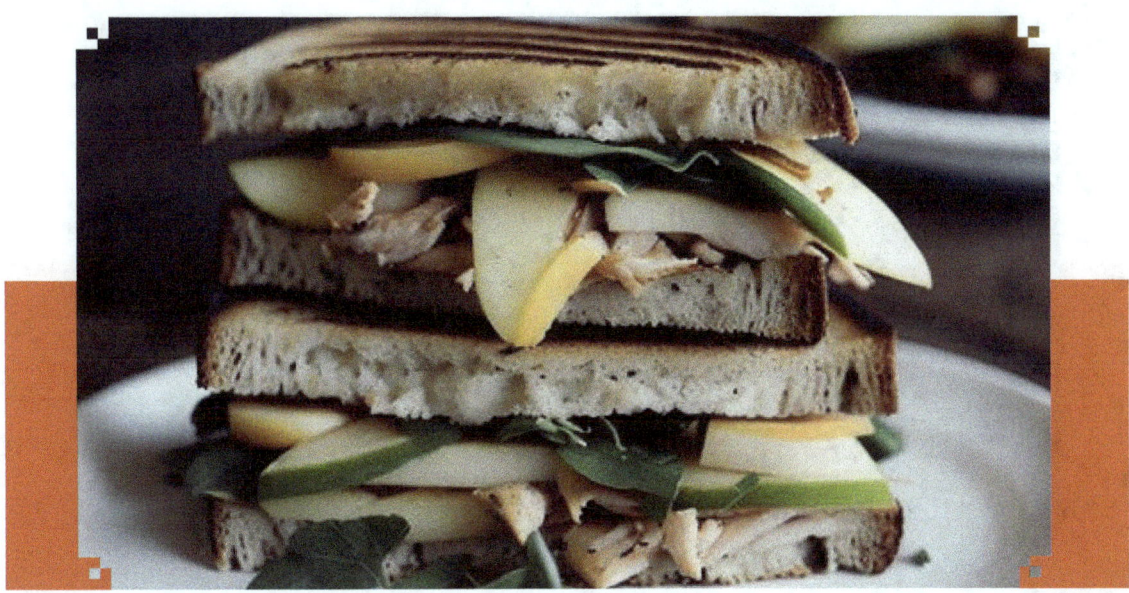

Chicken Pesto Pasta with Asparagus

Prep time: 10 minutes | Cook time: 10 minutes | Serves 2

- 2 oz. whole-wheat penne
- ½ cup shredded cooked chicken breast
- ½ container refrigerated basil pesto
- ¼ tsp. ground pepper
- ¼ oz. parmesan cheese, grated
- Small fresh basil leaves for garnish

1. Cook the pasta in a large pot according to package directions.
2. Return the pasta mixture to the pot. Stir in the chicken, pesto, salt, and pepper. Stir in the reserved cooking water 1 tbsp. at a time to reach the desired consistency.

PER SERVING

Calories: 422 | Protein: 31.4g | Carbs 32.2g | Fiber 0.8g | Fat: 18.4g

Toasted Chicken and Apple Sandwich

Prep time: 10 minutes | Cook time: 2 minutes | Serves 2

- 4 slices low-sodium multigrain bread
- 2 tablespoons low-fat mayonnaise
- 1 tart apple, cored and cut into thin slices
- 4 ounces cooked chicken breast, cut into 4 thin slices
- 1 cup gently packed shredded arugula

1. Toast bread until golden brown, and spread all four slices with mayonnaise.
2. Layer apple, chicken, and Cheddar cheese evenly on two slices of bread.
3. Top cheese with arugula and a second slice of toasted bread.
4. Cut sandwiches in half and serve.

PER SERVING

Calories: 432 | Fat: 17.6 g | Carbs: 40 g | Fiber: 4.4 g | Protein: 30.4 g

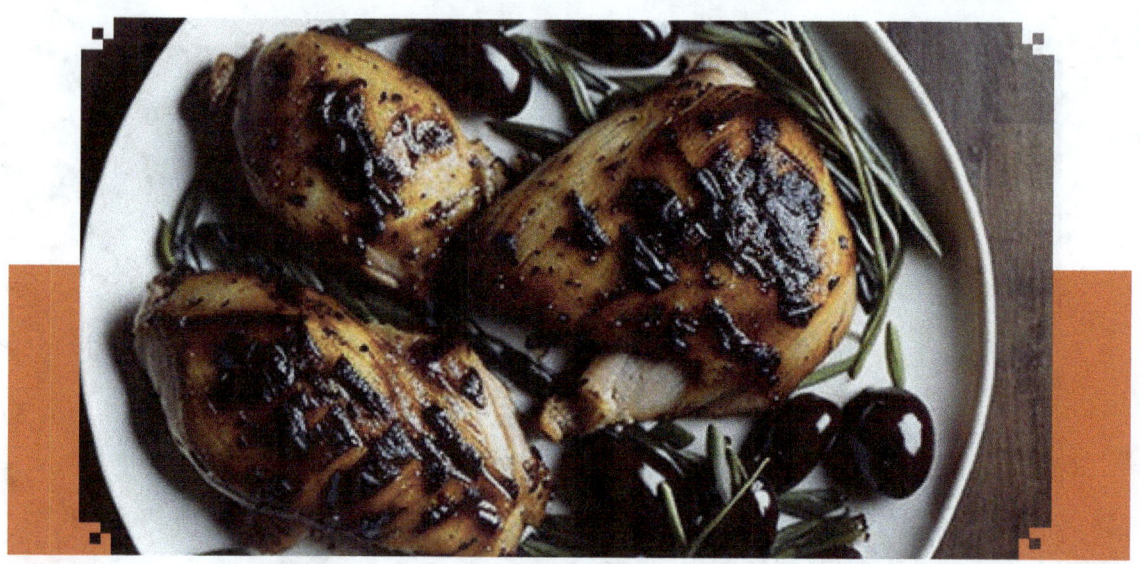

Fajita Chicken Wraps

Prep time: 10 minutes | Cook time: 6 minutes | Serves 2

- 12 ounces skinless chicken breast strips
- ½ teaspoon chili powder
- ¼ teaspoon garlic powder
- Non-stick cooking spray
- 1 red or green sweet pepper, seeded and cut into strips

1. Mix the chicken strips with the garlic powder and chili powder.
2. Add the chicken and sweet peppers. Cook for 6 minutes.
3. Toss in the ranch salad dressing.
4. Divide the mixture into warmed tortillas.
5. Top each tortilla with cheese and salsa.
6. Roll each tortilla and cut them in half.
7. Serve.

PER SERVING

Calories: 245 | Fat: 17g | Carbs: 8.7g | Fiber: 0g | Protein: 38.5g

Balsamic-Roasted Chicken Breasts

Prep time: 35 minutes | Cook time: 40 minutes | Serves 2

- ¼ cup balsamic vinegar
- 1 tablespoon olive oil
- 2 teaspoons dried oregano
- 2 garlic cloves, minced
- ⅛ teaspoon salt
- ½ teaspoon freshly ground black pepper
- cooking spray

1. In a small bowl, add the vinegar, olive oil, oregano, garlic, salt, and pepper. Mix to combine.
2. Preheat the oven to 400°F. Spray a small baking dish with cooking spray.
3. Let sit for 5 minutes, then serve with your favorite vegetables.

PER SERVING

Calories: 226 | Fat: 11g | Carbs: 6g | Fiber: 1g | Protein: 25g

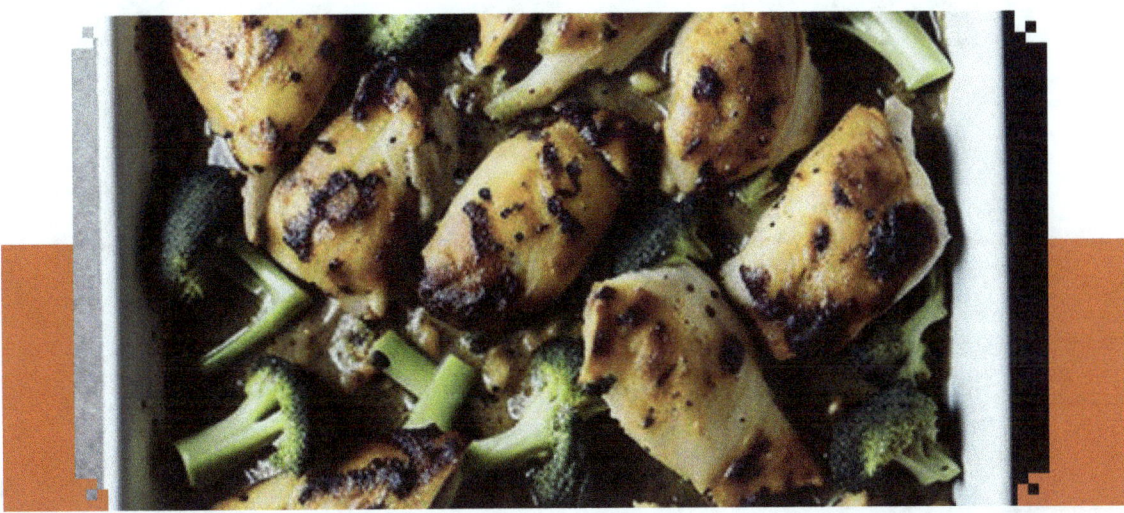

Bruschetta Chicken

Prep time: 8 minutes | Cook time: 12 minutes | Serves 2

For Chicken:
- 1½ teaspoon salt-free Italian seasoning
- ½ tablespoon olive oil
- 1 teaspoon garlic, minced

For Topping:
- 1½ garlic cloves, chopped finely
- 2 Roma tomatoes, chopped finely
- 1 tablespoon olive oil

For Chicken:
1. Take a bowl, add the chicken, garlic and Italian seasoning and mix them well altogether.
2. Remove the frying-pan from the heat and divide the chicken breasts onto serving plates.
3. Serve immediately.

PER SERVING

Calories: 234 | Fat: 13.7g | Carbs: 5.9g | Fiber: 1.8g | Protein: 22.9g

Chicken & Broccoli Casserole

Prep time: 10 minutes | Cook time: 35 minutes | Serves 2

- 1½ broccoli heads, cut into florets
- 2 tablespoons extra-virgin olive oil
- 2 garlic cloves, minced
- 2 skinless, boneless chicken thighs
- ½ teaspoon dried rosemary, crushed
- Fresh ground black pepper to taste

1. Preheat oven to 370° F and evenly grease a large baking dish.
2. Take a large bowl and add all the ingredients and toss to coat well.
3. Now, in the bottom of the dish arrange the broccoli florets and top it with chicken breasts in a single layer.
4. Bake it for about 35 minutes.
5. Serve hot and enjoy!

PER SERVING

Calories: 240 | Fat: 13.6g | Carbs: 4g | Fiber: 1.4g | Protein: 26.4g

Chapter 9

Meat Medley

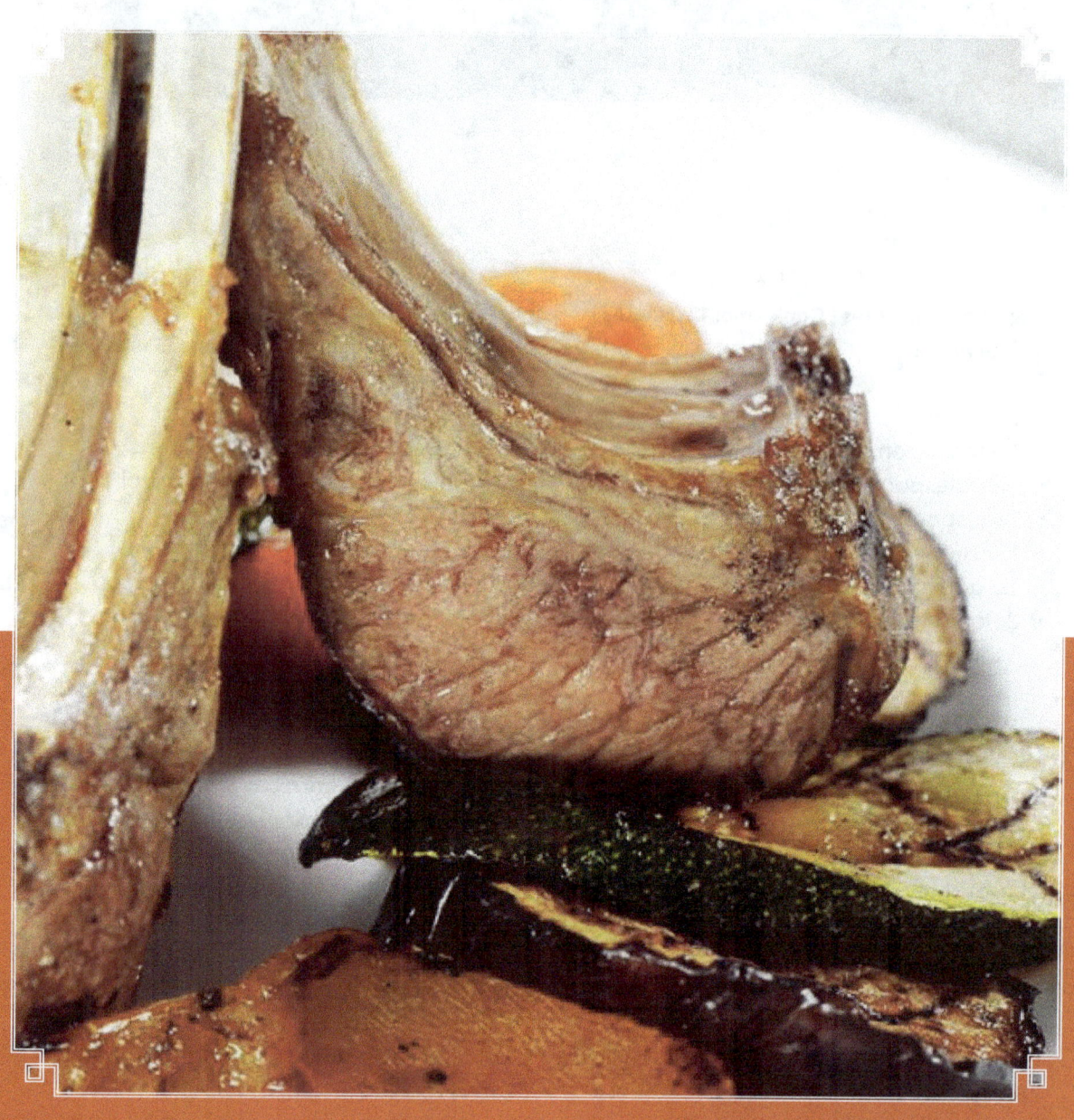

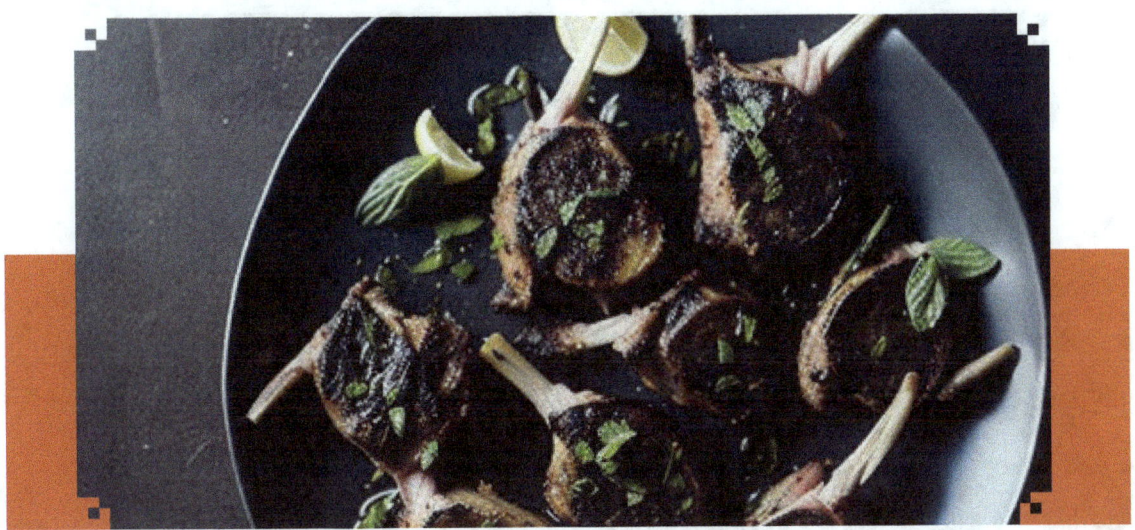

Beef Stroganoff

Prep time: 10 minutes | Cook time: 15 minutes | Serves 2

- ½ cup onion
- ½-pound boneless beef (fat removed)
- 4 cups yolkless egg noodles
- ½ can fat-free cream of mushroom
- ⅛ teaspoon white pepper
- ½ cup fat-free sour cream

1. Sauté the onions in a nonstick pan till the onions become translucent.
2. Add the beef into the pan and continue cooking till the beef turns brown and is tender.
3. Add the beef into this mixture as well, and once the mixture is warmed, remove it from heat.
4. Add the sour cream after removing it from heat.

PER SERVING

Calories: 391 | Fat: 23g | Carbs: 21g | Fiber: 1.3g | Protein: 25g

Mint and Garlic Marinated Lamb Chops

Prep time: 10 minutes | Cook time: 10 minutes | Serves 2

- 4 lamb loin chops
- 2 cloves garlic, minced
- 2 tablespoons fresh mint leaves, chopped
- 1 tablespoon olive oil
- 1 tablespoon lemon juice
- Salt and pepper to taste

1. In a shallow dish, combine minced garlic, chopped mint leaves, olive oil, lemon juice, salt, and pepper.
2. Add lamb chops to the dish and turn to coat evenly with the marinade. Let marinate for at least 30 minutes in the refrigerator.
3. Serve hot with a side of steamed vegetables or a fresh salad.

PER SERVING

Calories: 380|Fat: 28g|Carbs: 2g|Fiber: 0g|Protein: 30g

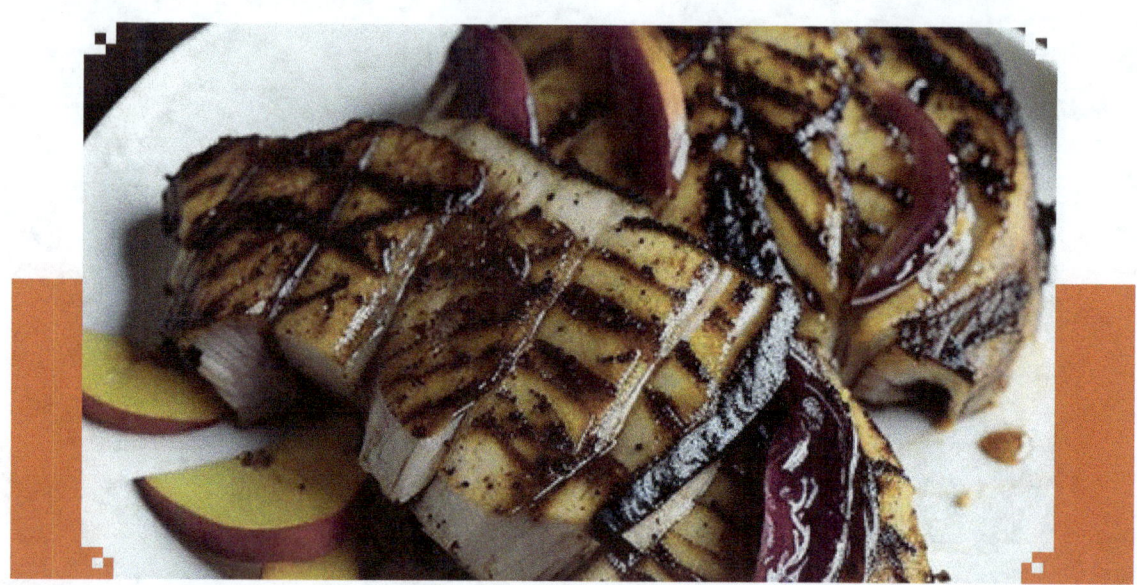

Pork Loin with Figgy Sauce

Prep time: 15 minutes | Cook time: 20 minutes | Serves 2

- 1 teaspoon dried rosemary
- 1 teaspoon dried thyme
- 1 teaspoon freshly ground pepper
- 2 garlic cloves, minced
- ½ cup dried figs, cut into quarters
- ½ cup white wine
- Juice of 1 lemon

1. Preheat the oven to 350°F. In a small bowl, mix the rosemary, thyme, and pepper to make a spice rub, and press into the pork loins.
2. While pork is resting, transfer the vegetables, figs, and pan juices into a blender. Process until smooth to make a gravy. Serve gravy with the pork.

PER SERVING

Calories: 386 | Fat: 14.3 g |Carbs: 27 g | Fiber: 4.1 g | Protein: 36 g

Apple-Cinnamon Baked Pork Chops

Prep time: 10 minutes | Cook time: 25 minutes | Serves 2

- 1 apple, peeled and sliced
- ½ teaspoon ground cinnamon
- freshly ground black pepper (optional)
- 2 tablespoons dark brown sugar
- ½ tablespoon extra-virgin olive oil

1. Preheat the oven to 375° F.
2. Layer the apples in the bottom of a casserole dish. Sprinkle with ½ teaspoon of the cinnamon.
3. Transfer to the oven and bake, uncovered, until an instant-read thermometer reads 145°F, 20 minutes. Allow to rest for 3 minutes before serving.

PER SERVING

Calories: 325 | Fat: 16 g | Carbs: 24 g | Fiber: 3 g | Protein: 24 g

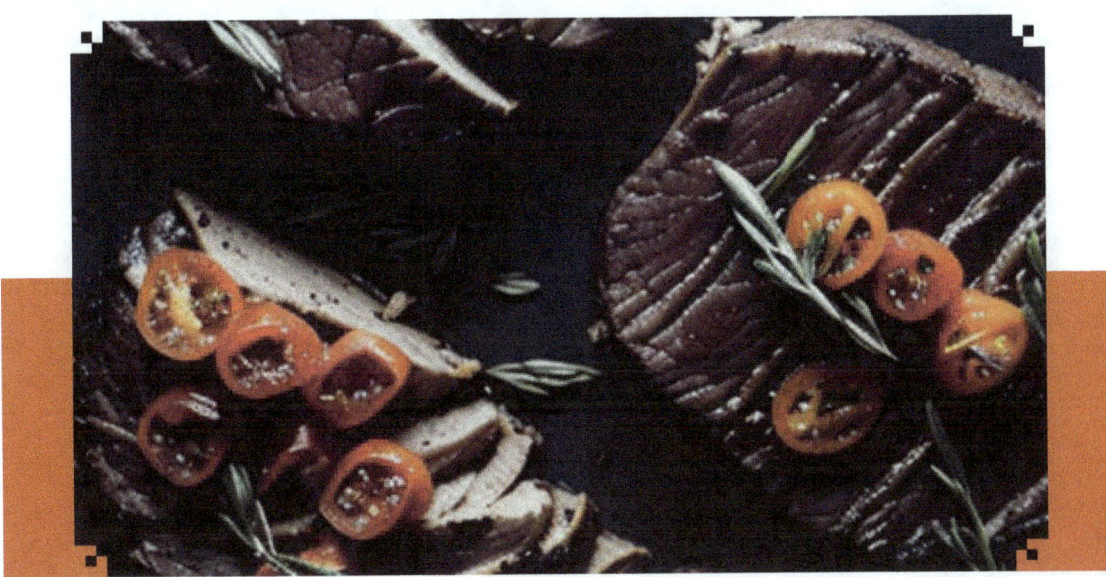

Mushroom and Red Wine Braised Beef

Prep time: 15 minutes | Cook time: 2 hours | Serves 2

- 1 lb beef chuck roast, cut into chunks
- 1 onion, chopped
- 2 cloves garlic, minced
- 1 teaspoon dried thyme
- Salt and pepper to taste

1. Preheat oven to 325°F (160°C).
2. In a Dutch oven or oven-safe pot, heat olive oil over medium heat.
3. Add chopped onion and minced garlic, sauté until softened.
4. Braise for about 1.5 to 2 hours, or until the beef is tender.
5. Serve hot with mashed potatoes or whole grain rice.

PER SERVING

Calories: 450| Fat: 22g| Carbs: 10g| Fiber: 2g| Protein: 40g

Beef Tenderloin with Balsamic Tomatoes

Prep time: 5 minutes | Cook time: 20 minutes | Serves 2

- ½ cup balsamic vinegar
- ¾ cup coarsely chopped, seeded tomato
- 2 teaspoons olive oil
- 1 teaspoon fresh thyme (or ½ teaspoon dried)

1. In a small saucepan, bring the balsamic vinegar to a boil. Reduce the heat and simmer, uncovered, for 5 ¼ cup. Stir in the tomatoes and cook for 1 to 2 minutes more. Remove the saucepan from the heat.
2. Spoon the balsamic tomatoes over the steaks, and sprinkle with the thyme. Serve immediately.

PER SERVING

Calories: 298 | Fat: 20g | Carbs: 11g | Fiber: 1g | Protein: 17g

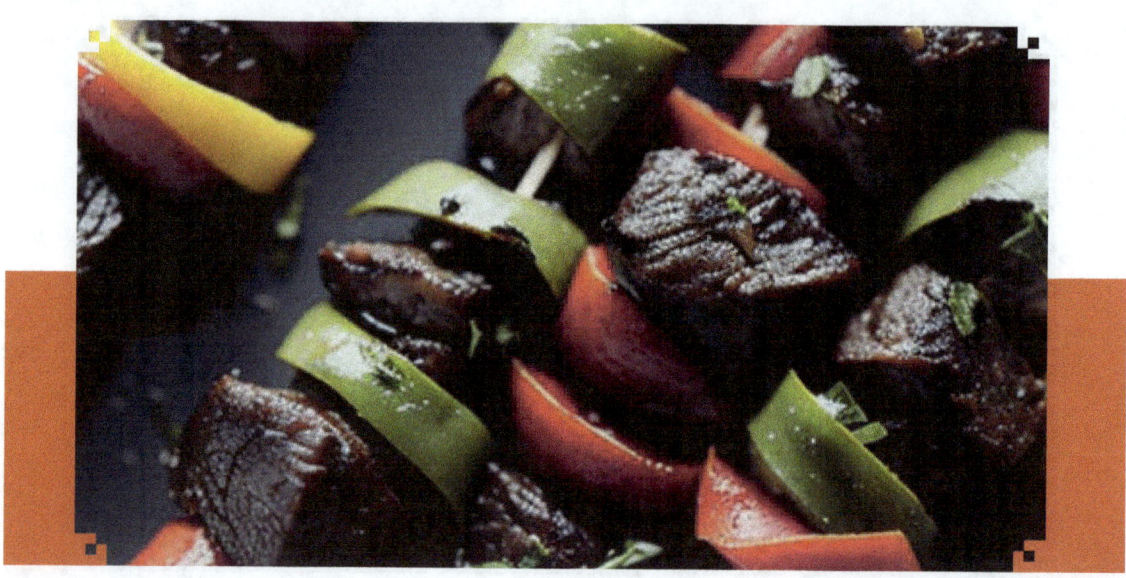

Orange-Beef Stir-Fry

Prep time: 10 minutes | Cook time: 10 minutes | Serves 2

- 1 tablespoon cornstarch
- ¼ cup cold water
- ¼ cup orange juice
- 1 tablespoon reduced-sodium soy sauce
- 2 teaspoons olive oil, divided
- 3 cups frozen stir-fry vegetable blend
- 1 garlic clove, minced

1. In a small bowl, mix the cornstarch, water, orange juice, and soy sauce until smooth. Set the mixture aside.
2. In a large wok or skillet, heat 1 teaspoon of olive oil over medium-high heat. Stir-fry the beef for 3 to 4 minutes, until no longer pink. Remove to a plate or bowl and cover to keep warm.

PER SERVING

Calories: 268 | Fat: 10g | Carbs: 8g | Fiber: 3g | Protein: 26g

Lemon Herb Beef Kabobs

Prep time: 15 minutes | Cook time: 10 minutes | Serves 2

- 8 ounces beef sirloin, cut into cubes
- 1 bell pepper, cut into chunks
- 1 red onion, cut into chunks
- 2 tablespoons olive oil
- 1 tablespoon fresh lemon juice
- 1 teaspoon dried thyme
- 1 teaspoon dried rosemary
- Salt and pepper to taste

1. In a bowl, combine olive oil, lemon juice, dried thyme, dried rosemary, salt, and pepper.
2. Thread beef cubes, bell pepper chunks, and red onion chunks onto skewers.
3. Serve hot with a side of whole grains or roasted vegetables.

PER SERVING

Calories: 350| Fat: 20g| Carbs: 8g| Fiber: 2g| Protein: 35g

Chapter 10

Veggie Venture

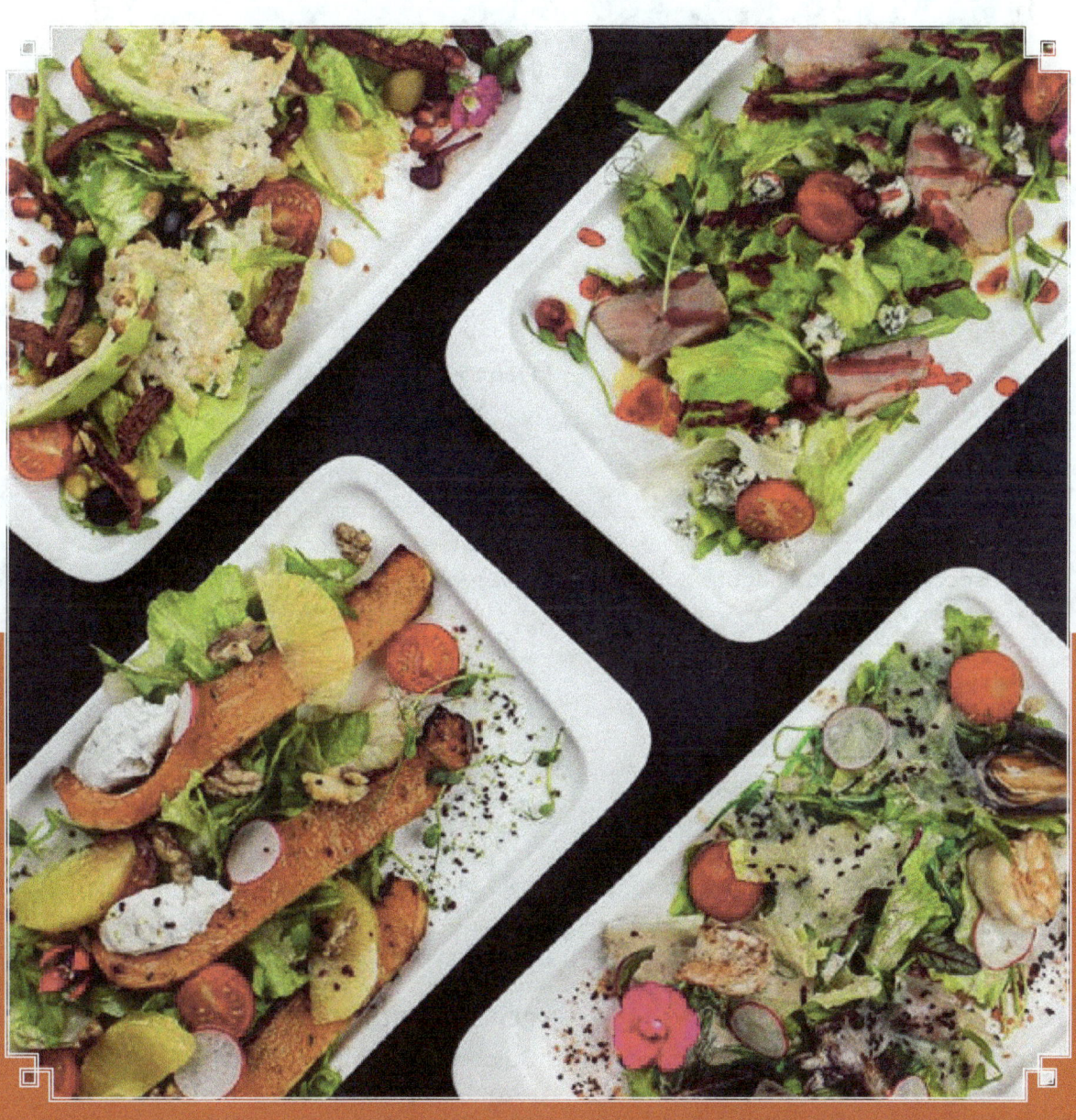

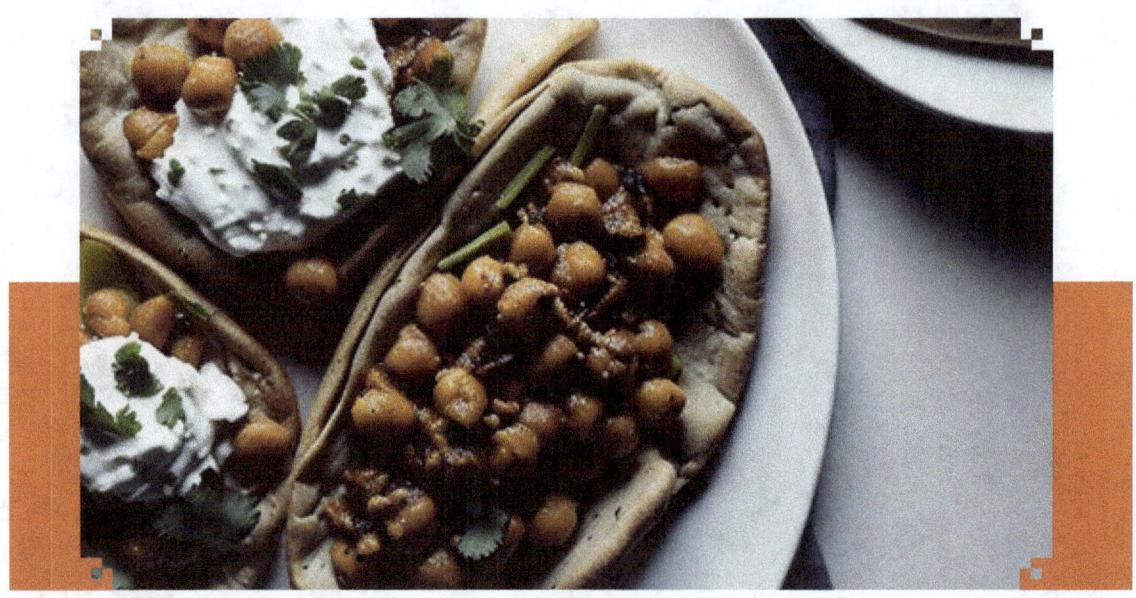

Sautéed Spinach with Pumpkin Seeds

Prep time: 5 minutes |Cook time: 15 minutes |Serves 2

- 2 tablespoons raw shelled pumpkin seeds
- 2 teaspoons extra-virgin olive oil
- 1 teaspoon balsamic vinegar
- 1 teaspoon water
- 1 bunch spinach, large stems removed
- freshly ground black pepper

1. Preheat the oven to 350 °F.
2. Spread the pumpkin seeds on a r Remove from the pan to cool.
3. Transfer to a serving dish, and sprinkle with the toasted pumpkin seeds and goat cheese. Top with black pepper, if desired.

PER SERVING:

Calories: 136| Fat: 11g| Carbs: 5g| Protein: 7g | Fiber: 5g

Chickpea Gyros

Prep time: 5 minutes | Cook time: 5 minutes | Serves 2

- 1 tablespoon extra-virgin olive oil
- 1 (15-ounce) can low-sodium chickpeas, drained and rinsed
- ½ teaspoon cayenne pepper
- 2 whole-wheat pita rounds
- ¼ cup Tzatziki

1. In a large skillet, heat the oil over medium heat.
2. Add the chickpeas, and sauté for 2 to 3 minutes, or until heated through.
3. Sprinkle with the paprika and cayenne. Mix well. Cook for 30 seconds, or until fragrant. Remove from the heat.
4. Top with the tzatziki.

PER SERVING

Calories: 168 | Fat: 6g | Carbs: 23g | Fiber: 5g | Protein: 6g

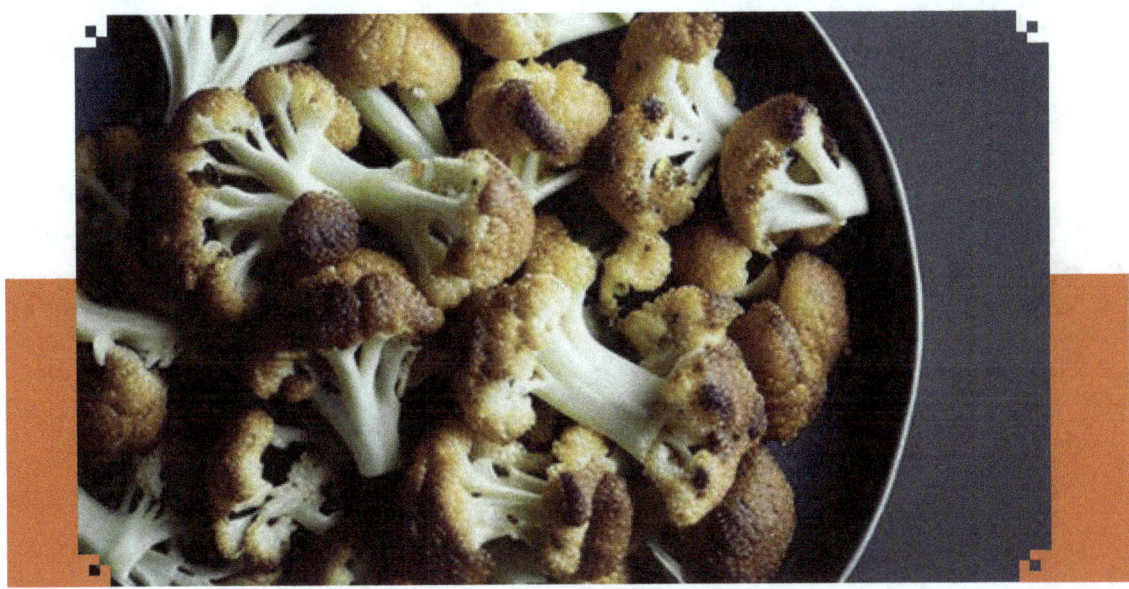

Roasted Eggplant with Tahini-Garlic Dressing

Prep time: 10 minutes | Cook time: 20 minutes | Serves 2

- ¼ teaspoon smoked paprika
- 1 teaspoon avocado oil
- 2 small eggplants, cut into bite-size pieces
- ¼ cup Tahini-Garlic Dressing

1. Preheat the oven to 425°F. Line a baking sheet with parchment paper.
2. Evenly coat the eggplant with the paprika and oil. Spread the eggplant on the prepared baking sheet.
3. Add the eggplant to the dressing and toss to coat. Divide into appropriate portions and serve, or store in the refrigerator for 3 to 4 days.

PER SERVING

Calories: 264 | Fat: 15g | Carbs: 33g | Sugars: 16g | Fiber: 15g | Protein: 7g

Life-Changing Roasted Cauliflower

Prep time: 10 minutes | Cook time: 30 minutes | Serves 2

- 1 (12-ounce) bag frozen cauliflower florets (about 3 cups)
- 2 tablespoons canola or sunflower oil
- ¼ teaspoon kosher salt
- ½ teaspoon ground cumin (optional)
- freshly ground black pepper (optional)

1. Preheat the oven to 420°F. Line a rimmed baking sheet with parchment paper.
2. Roast the cauliflower for about 25 minutes, tossing every 10 minutes so it cooks evenly. Don't worry if it gets dark brown in spots—that's the best part.

PER SERVING

Calories: 166 | Fat: 15g | Carbs: 8g | Fiber: 4g | Protein: 3g

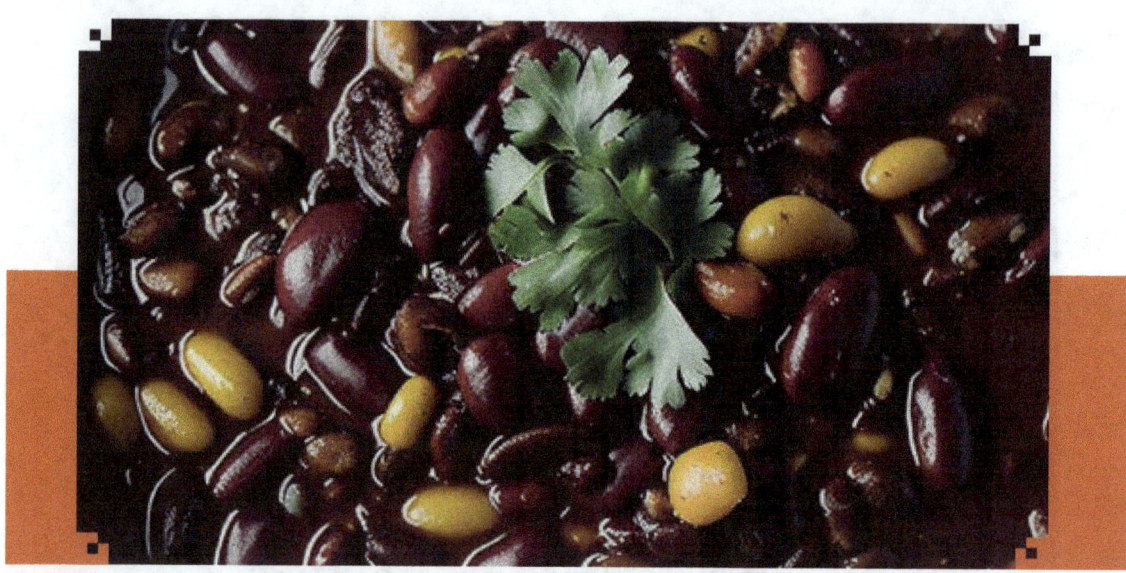

Caramelized Onions

Prep time: 5 minutes | Cook time: 15 minutes | Serves 2

- 2 tablespoons extra virgin olive oil
- 4 cups, thinly sliced white onions
- 1 teaspoon brown sugar
- 1/8 teaspoon cracked black pepper

1. Heat a medium-sized saucepan over medium heat. Add the oil and when the oil is hot, add the onions, and then the sugar and pepper. Sauté for 5 to 10 minutes, stirring constantly to avoid burning. Once the onions are translucent and start turning brown, cover the pan and turn the heat down to low.
2. Let the onions "sweat" for about 5 more minutes. When done, they should be dark brown and very soft.

PER SERVING

Calories:43 | Fat:3 g | Carbs:5 g | Fiber:.08 g |Protein:.05 g

Spicy Bean Chili

Prep time: 10 minutes | Cook time: 20 minutes | Serves 2

- 1 teaspoon of grapeseed oil
- ½ medium size red onion
- ½ Jalapeno pepper
- 1 garlic clove
- 15 ounces of low sodium red kidney beans
- ¼ teaspoon of sea salt
- ⅛ teaspoon of ground cinnamon

1. Warm oil in a saucepan with medium-high heat.
2. Add the onion and Jalapeño, after which you sauté for 5 minutes till the onion is caramelized.
3. Put the garlic and sauté until fragrant for about 30 seconds.
4. Enjoy.

PER SERVING

Calories: 270 | Fat: 2g | Carbs: 45g | Fiber: 17g | Protein: 17g

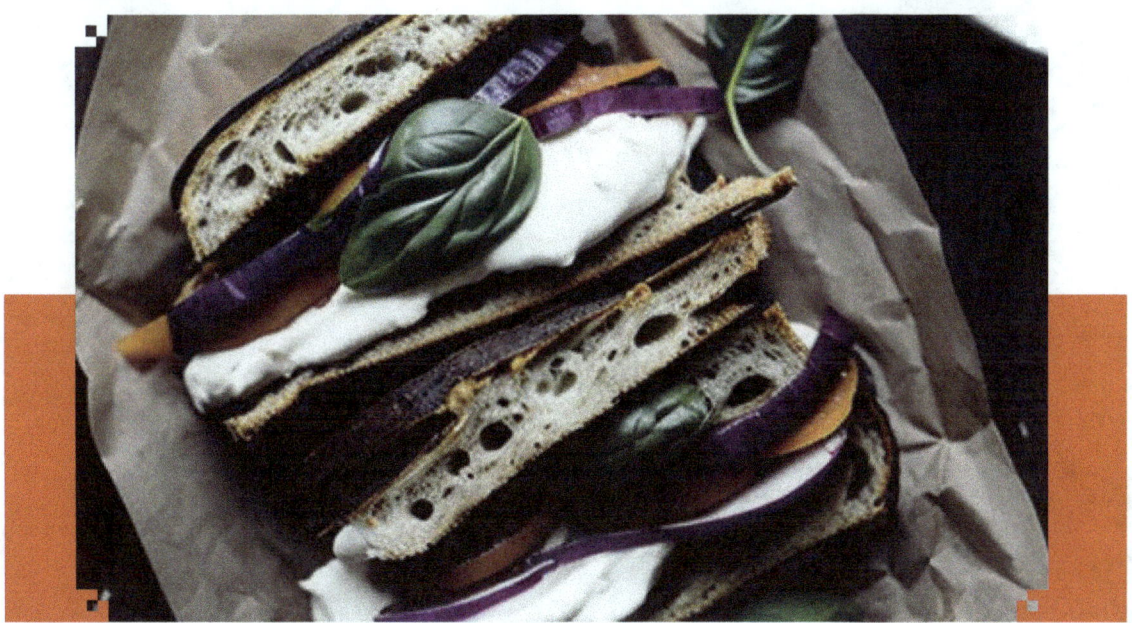

Basil Tomato Crostini

Prep time: 10 minutes | Cook time: none | Serves 2

- 4 plum tomatoes, chopped
- ¼ cup minced fresh basil
- 2 teaspoons olive oil
- 1 garlic clove, minced
- Freshly ground pepper
- ¼ pound Italian bread, cut into 4 slices and toasted

1. Toss the tomatoes with the oil, garlic, pepper, and basil in a bowl.
2. Cover and allow them to sit for 30 minutes.
3. Top the toast slices with the mixture.
4. Serve.

PER SERVING

Calories: 104 | Fat: 3.5g | Carbs: 15g | Fiber: 0.4g | Protein: 2g

Roasted Eggplant Sandwiches

Prep time: 10 minutes | Cook time: 30 minutes | Serves 2

- Nonstick cooking spray (optional)
- ¼ teaspoon freshly ground black pepper
- 1 tomato, sliced
- 1 small red onion, sliced
- ½ cup chopped fresh basil
- 4 whole wheat bread slices

1. Preheat the oven to 375°F. Line a sheet pan with aluminum foil or coat with nonstick cooking spray.
2. Brush both sides of the eggplant with skin is wrinkly and the eggplant is soft and let cool.

PER SERVING

Calories: 542 | Fat: 24g | Carbs: 56g | Fiber: 9g | Protein: 21g

Chapter 11

Sweet Finale

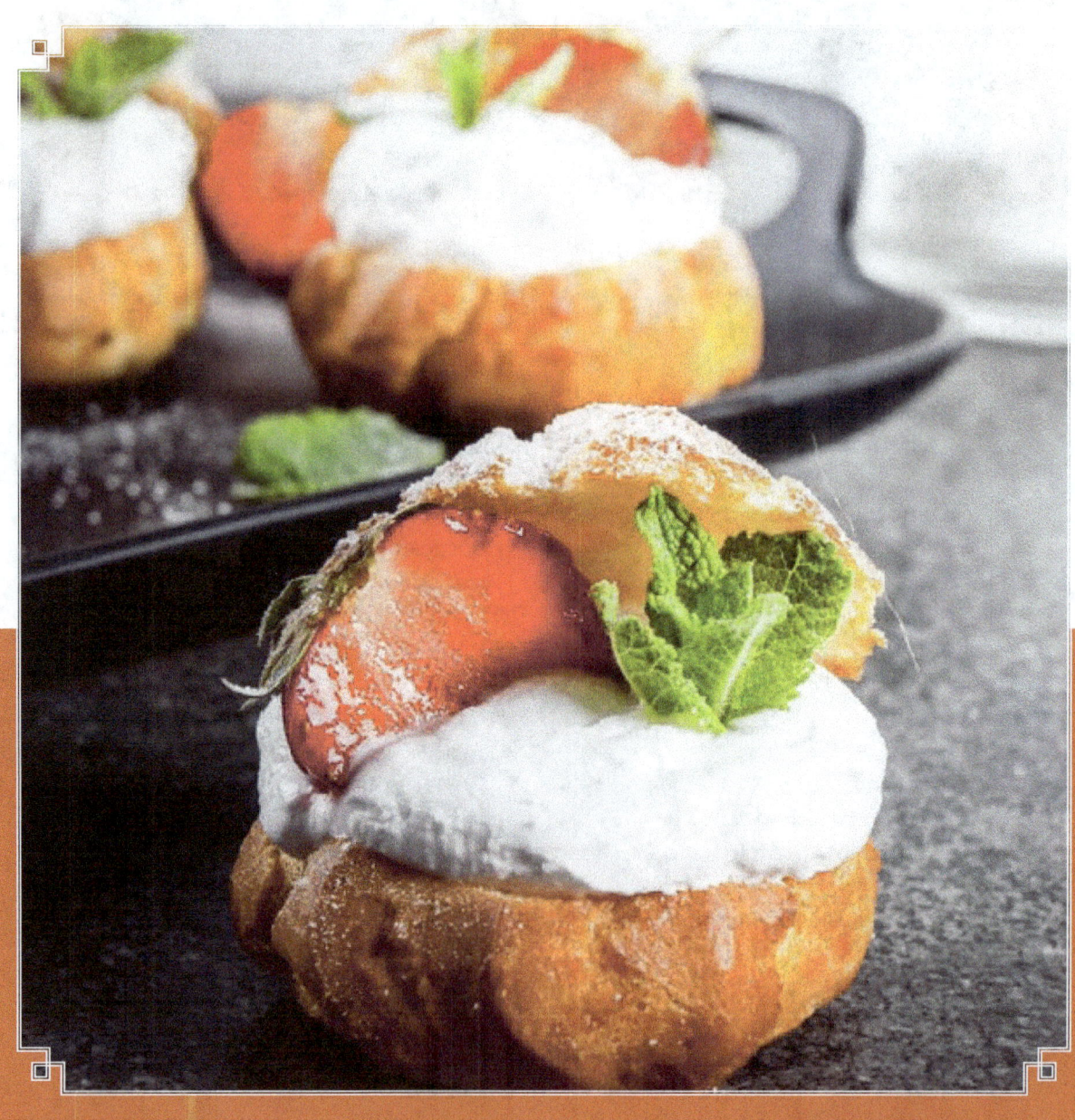

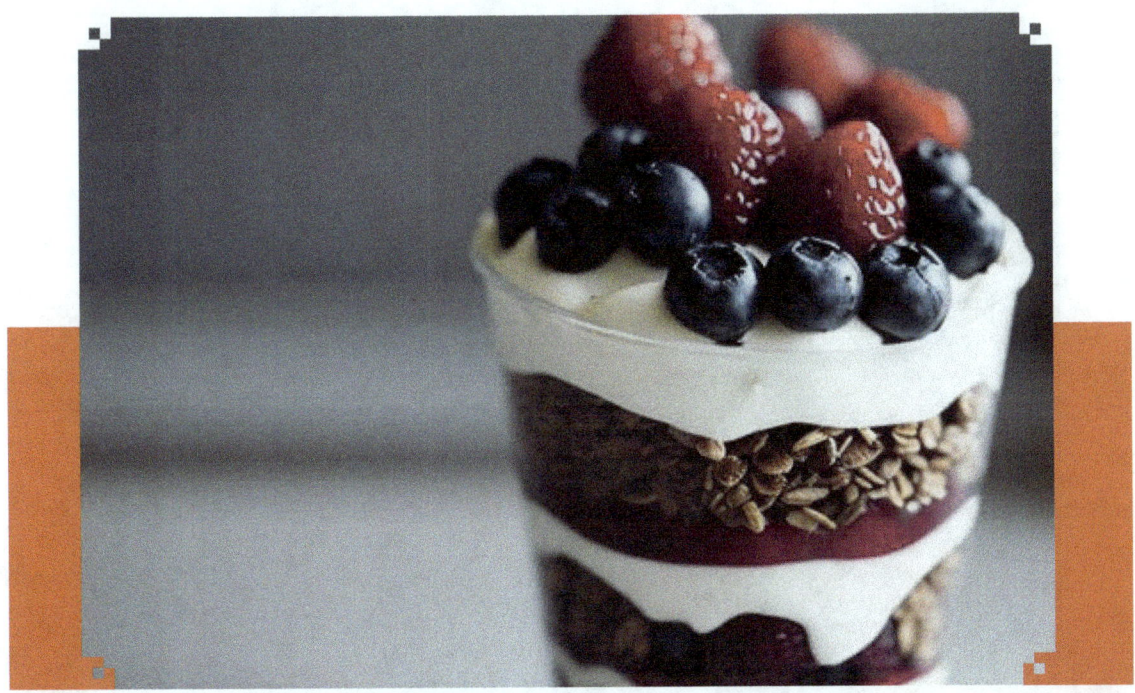

Raspberry-Lime Sorbet

Prep time: 5 minutes | Cook time: 10 minutes, plus 2 to 4 hours to chill | Serves 2

- 2 cups frozen raspberries
- 2 teaspoons honey
- 1 teaspoon lime juice
- ½ cup warm water

1. In a blender, blend the raspberries, honey, lime juice, and water on high for 2 to 3 minutes until well combined.
2. Place the mixture in a freezer-safe cup or in a ice-pop mold. Freeze 2 to 4 hours until firm. Store in the freezer in an airtight container for up to 1 month.

PER SERVING

Calories: 162 | Fat: 2g | Carbs: 37g | Fiber: 11g | Protein: 3g

Fresh Berry Parfait

Prep time: 10 minutes | Cook time: none | Serves 2

- 1 cup low-fat Greek yogurt
- 2 tablespoons honey or maple syrup
- 1/4 cup granola
- Fresh mint leaves for garnish (optional)

1. In two serving glasses, layer Greek yogurt, mixed berries, and granola.
2. Drizzle honey or maple syrup over each parfait.
3. Repeat layering until glasses are filled.
4. Serve immediately or refrigerate until ready to serve.

PER SERVING

Calories: 250| Fat: 3g| Carbs: 45g| Fiber: 6g| Protein: 14g

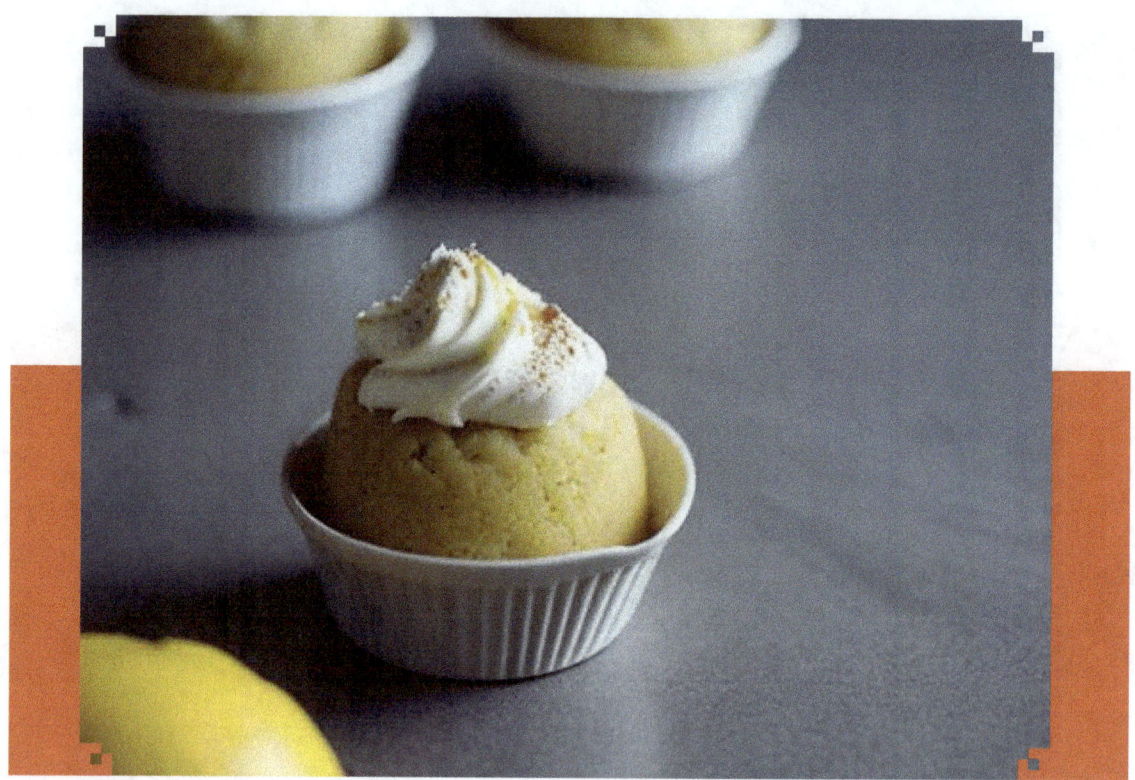

Frozen Mango Treat

Prep time: 5 minutes | Cook time: none | Serves 2

- 1½ cup frozen mangoes, peeled and chopped
- ½ tablespoon fresh mint leaves
- 1 tablespoon fresh lime juice
- ¼ cup chilled water

1. Add all the ingredients in a blender and blend well.
2. Take out and refrigerate for about two hours.
3. Serve and enjoy!

PER SERVING

Calories: 278 | Fat: 1.7g | Carbs: 69.9g | Fiber: 7.5g | Protein: 3.9g

Lemon Pudding Cakes

Prep time: 15 minutes | Cook time: 40 minutes | Serves 2

- 2 eggs
- ¼ teaspoon salt
- ¾ cup sugar
- 1 cup skim milk
- 1 tablespoon finely grated lemon peel
- 1 tablespoon melted butter

1. Preheat the oven to 350°F.
2. Grease two custard cups with cooking oil.
3. Serve.

PER SERVING

Calories: 182 | Fat: 6g | Carbs: 15g | Fiber: 2g | Protein: 1.2g

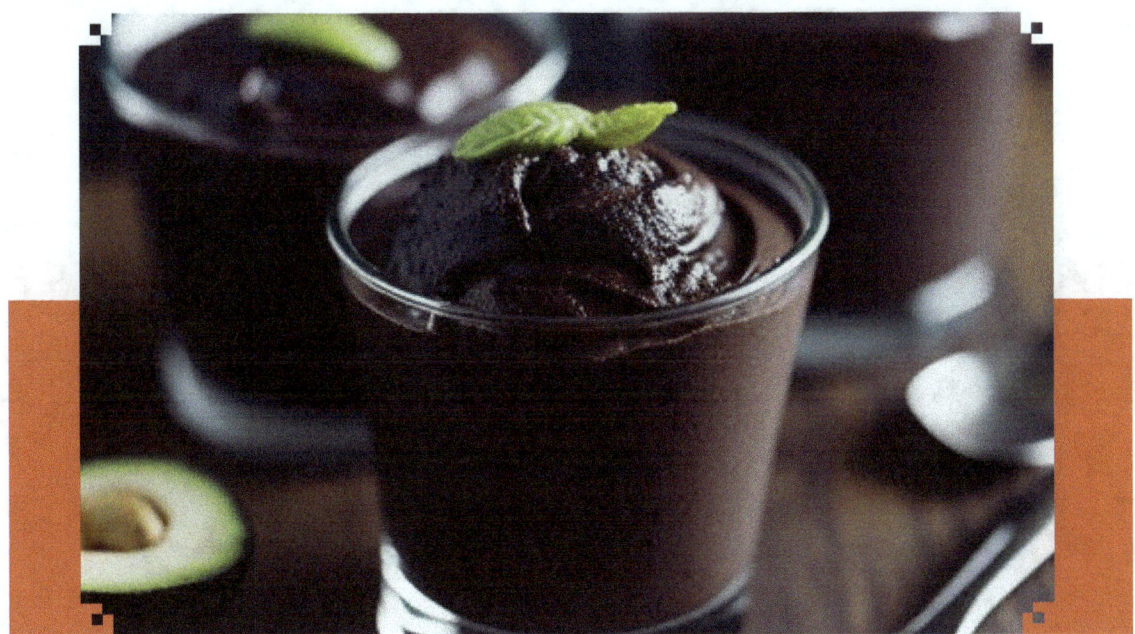

Chocolate-Covered Strawberry Smoothie

Prep time: 5 minutes | Cook time: 10 minutes | Serves 2

- 1 to 2 cups ice
- 1 cup nonfat or low-fat milk
- ¾ cup plain nonfat or low-fat greek yogurt
- 1 cup frozen strawberries
- 1 frozen banana, peeled and sliced
- 2 tablespoons unsweetened cocoa powder
- ½ teaspoon vanilla extract
- 1 teaspoon honey (optional)

1. In a blender, combine all of the ingredients, and blend until smooth.
2. Pour into two tall glasses and enjoy immediately.

PER SERVING

Calories: 181 | Fat: 1g | Carbs: 33g | Fiber: 5g | Protein: 15g

Dark Chocolate Avocado Mousse

Prep time: 10 minutes | Cook time: none | Serves 2

- 1 ripe avocado, peeled and pitted
- 1/4 cup unsweetened cocoa powder
- 1/4 cup almond milk (or any milk of choice)
- 2 tablespoons honey or maple syrup
- Fresh berries for garnish (optional)

1. In a blender or food processor, combine avocado, cocoa powder, almond milk, honey or maple syrup, vanilla extract, and a pinch of salt.
2. Refrigerate for at least 30 minutes before serving.
3. Garnish with fresh berries if desired.

PER SERVING

Calories: 250| Fat: 15g| Carbs: 30g| Fiber: 10g| Protein: 4g

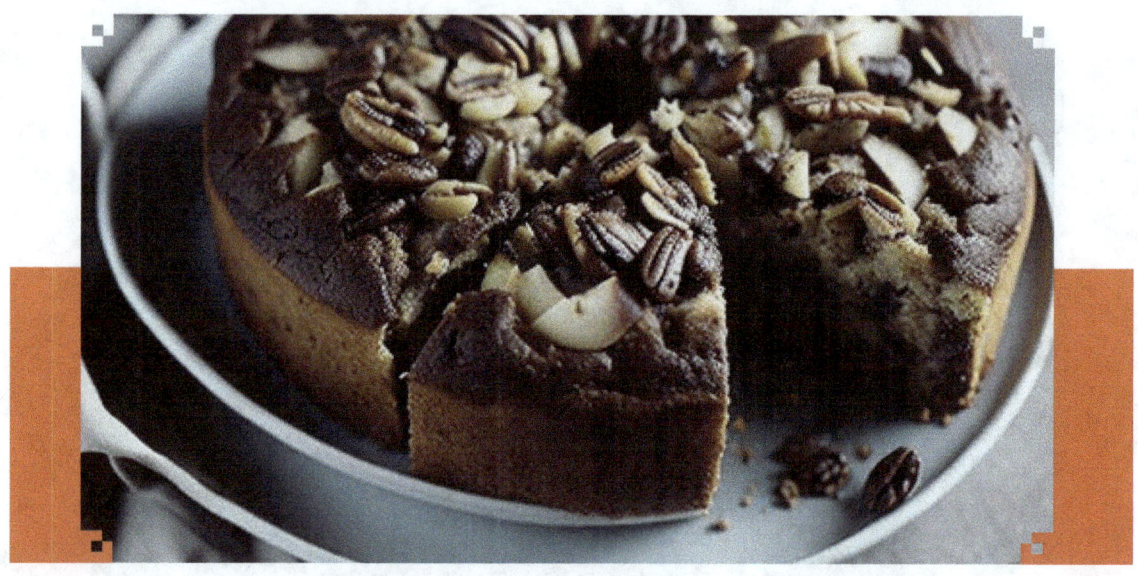

Mini Banana Split

Prep time: 5 minutes | Cook time: none | Serves 2

- 3 tablespoons dark chocolate chips or chopped dark chocolate
- 1 large banana, sliced
- 1 cup low-fat frozen yogurt
- 1/4 cup chopped strawberries
- 1/4 cup chopped pineapple
- 2 tablespoons toasted chopped almonds

1. Place the chocolate in a small, microwave-safe bowl, and microwave for 10 seconds. Stir the chocolate, and repeat the process until the chocolate is fully melted.
2. Assemble banana splits in two small ramekins by arranging banana slices Add the toppings, and drizzle each with chocolate.

PER SERVING

Calories:332 | Fat:11 g | Carbs:58 g | Fiber:5 g | Protein:6 g

Apple Coffee Cake

Prep time: 5 minutes | Cook time: 30 minutes | Serves 2

- 1 cup tart apples, cored, peeled, chopped
- 1/4 cup dark raisins
- 1/2 cup all-purpose flour, sifted
- 1/2 teaspoon ground cinnamon
- 1/4 teaspoon baking soda

1. Preheat the oven to 350°F.
2. Lightly oil a small baking dish or cake pan (such as an 8x4-inch loaf pan).
3. In a mixing bowl, combine the apples with sugar, raisins, and pecans. Mix well and let it stand for 30 minutes.
4. Bake for 30 to 35 minutes or until a toothpick inserted into the center comes out clean.
5. Cool the cake slightly before serving.

PER SERVING:

Calories: 196| Fat: 8g| Fiber: 2g| Protein: 3g| Carbs: 31g

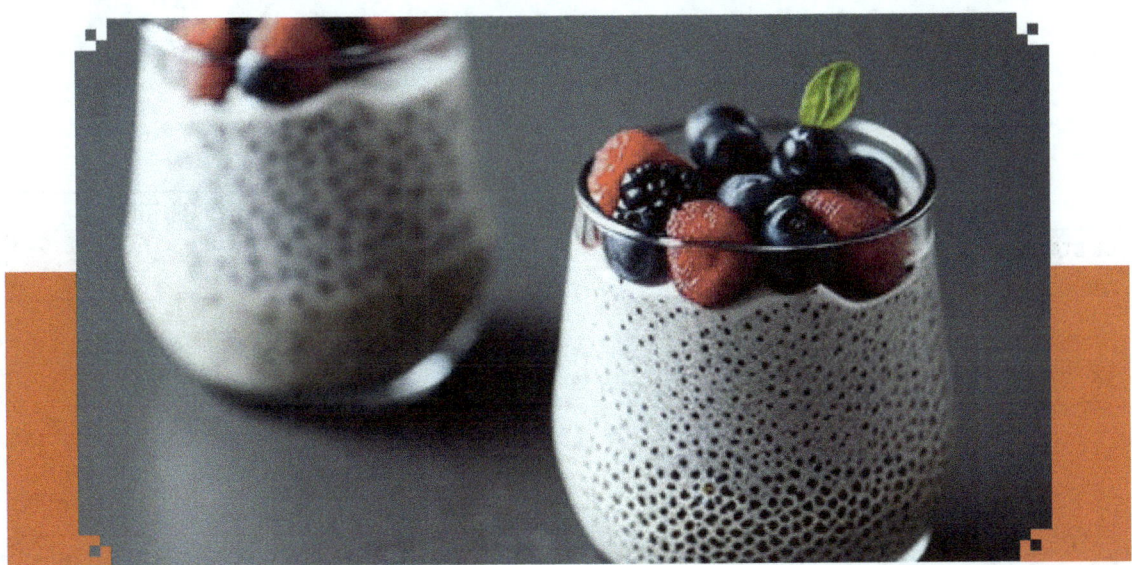

Cashew Cream Mousse

Prep time: 50 minutes | Cook time: none | Serves 2

- ½ cup cashews, presoaked
- 1 tablespoon honey
- 1 teaspoon vanilla extract
- 1 large banana, sliced (reserve 4 slices for garnish)
- 1 cup plain non-fat Greek yogurt

1. Place the cashews in a small bowl and cover with 1 cup of water.
2. Soak at room temperature for 2 to 3 hours. Drain, rinse and set aside.
3. Fold in yogurt, mix well. Cover. Chill in the refrigerator, covered, for at least 45 minutes.
4. Portion mousse into two serving bowls.
5. Enjoy.

PER SERVING

Calories: 329 | Fat: 14 g | Carbs: 37 g | Fiber: 3 g | Protein: 17 g

Chia Seed Pudding

Prep time: 5 minutes | Cook time: 5 minutes | Serves 2

- 1/4 cup chia seeds
- 1 cup unsweetened almond milk (or any milk of choice)
- 1 tablespoon honey or maple syrup
- 1/2 teaspoon vanilla extract
- Fresh fruit for topping (such as berries, sliced banana)

1. In a mixing bowl, whisk together chia seeds, almond milk, honey or maple syrup, and vanilla extract.
2. Let the mixture sit for 5 minutes, then whisk again to prevent clumping.
3. Divide the pudding into two serving dishes and top with fresh fruit before serving.

PER SERVING

Calories: 180| Fat: 9g| Carbs: 22g| Fiber: 11g| Protein: 5g

Appendix 1 Measurement Conversion Chart

Volume Equivalents (Dry)

US STANDARD	METRIC (APPROXIMATE)
1/8 teaspoon	0.5 mL
1/4 teaspoon	1 mL
1/2 teaspoon	2 mL
3/4 teaspoon	4 mL
1 teaspoon	5 mL
1 tablespoon	15 mL
1/4 cup	59 mL
1/2 cup	118 mL
3/4 cup	177 mL
1 cup	235 mL
2 cups	475 mL
3 cups	700 mL
4 cups	1 L

Volume Equivalents (Liquid)

US STANDARD	US STANDARD (OUNCES)	METRIC (AP-PROXIMATE)
2 tablespoons	1 fl.oz.	30 mL
1/4 cup	2 fl.oz.	60 mL
1/2 cup	4 fl.oz.	120 mL
1 cup	8 fl.oz.	240 mL
1 1/2 cup	12 fl.oz.	355 mL
2 cups or 1 pint	16 fl.oz.	475 mL
4 cups or 1 quart	32 fl.oz.	1 L
1 gallon	128 fl.oz.	4 L

Temperatures Equivalents

FAHRENHEIT(F)	CELSIUS(C) APPROXIMATE)
225 °F	107 °C
250 °F	120 ° °C
275 °F	135 °C
300 °F	150 °C
325 °F	160 °C
350 °F	180 °C
375 °F	190 °C
400 °F	205 °C
425 °F	220 °C
450 °F	235 °C
475 °F	245 °C
500 °F	260 °C

Weight Equivalents

US STANDARD	METRIC (APPROXIMATE)
1 ounce	28 g
2 ounces	57 g
5 ounces	142 g
10 ounces	284 g
15 ounces	425 g
16 ounces (1 pound)	455 g
1.5 pounds	680 g
2 pounds	907 g

Appendix 2 The Dirty Dozen and Clean Fifteen

The Environmental Working Group (EWG) is a nonprofit, nonpartisan organization dedicated to protecting human health and the environment Its mission is to empower people to live healthier lives in a healthier environment. This organization publishes an annual list of the twelve kinds of produce, in sequence, that have the highest amount of pesticide residue-the Dirty Dozen-as well as a list of the fifteen kinds ofproduce that have the least amount of pesticide residue-the Clean Fifteen.

THE DIRTY DOZEN

The 2016 Dirty Dozen includes the following produce. These are considered among the year's most important produce to buy organic:

Strawberries	Spinach
Apples	Tomatoes
Nectarines	Bell peppers
Peaches	Cherry tomatoes
Celery	Cucumbers
Grapes	Kale/collard greens
Cherries	Hot peppers

The Dirty Dozen list contains two additional itemskale/collard greens and hot peppers-because they tend to contain trace levels of highly hazardous pesticides.

THE CLEAN FIFTEEN

The least critical to buy organically are the Clean Fifteen list. The following are on the 2016 list:

Avocados	Papayas
Corn	Kiw
Pineapples	Eggplant
Cabbage	Honeydew
Sweet peas	Grapefruit
Onions	Cantaloupe
Asparagus	Cauliflower
Mangos	

Some of the sweet corn sold in the United States are made from genetically engineered (GE) seedstock. Buy organic varieties of these crops to avoid GE produce.

Appendix 3 Index

Polly R. Pendleton

Printed in the USA
CPSIA information can be obtained
at www.ICGtesting.com
CBHW070402120624
9795CB00019B/15